MERCURY POISONING
AND DEEP FAITH

MERCURY POISONING AND DEEP FAITH

Pamela Elizabeth Lacek, R.N.

To order additional copies of this book, contact:

Pamela E. Lacek, R.N.
R N Healing Arts
1-519-401-2324
www.rnhealingarts.com
placek@rnhealingarts.com

Xlibris Corporation
1-888-795-4274
www.Xlibris.com
Orders@Xlibris.com
31526

CONTENTS

DEDICATION

I thank the Father, Son, Holy Spirit and Mother Mary for their guidance and blessings and the kind people that they drew into my life.

INTRODUCTION

The author tells her story with both biting and heart warming candor. And through the paradox of a self-disclosing vulnerability she demonstrates the invulnerability of an indomitable spirit, which has grown strong through private pain.

She places her personal circumstances, along with her inner life, thoughts, and emotions, right on the page for all to see, and carries the reader through a range of emotions—from anger, disappointment, and frustration, through to faith, hope, and love, and a clear sense of humor and joie de vivre. These latter arise from an intense spiritual sensitivity and core devotion to the centre of her faith, Jesus Christ, and His sacrificial death on the Cross for her.

Her latest work is all of these: An unusual, a tragic, and a triumphant, story. It is her story, and it is still unfolding.

Peter A. Black, freelance writer

CHAPTER 1
The Beginning

I'll start with the year 2001. This is the year that I felt like a simple it, not a person. I had transient numbness and hip displacement. Libido was non-existent, I couldn't even cry when I felt emotional turmoil inside. I so desperately needed a menstrual cycle to give some order to my life. People have no idea of the beauty in a menstrual cycle. It's a rhythm. I felt like an ocean without the ebb and flow of the tides. There was no time for release of feelings or appreciation of womanhood. I suppose that is in part what singing has brought back to me. I'm talking about womanhood and release of feelings. I have no menstrual cycle yet; well I say this at the time I wrote this part anyhow. It has brought me love of self because of the redemption of a gift given to me by God.

Finally someone besides me noticed that I love to sing and have a voice. But then again, I asked God for a favor. I asked that if my son Daniel could be free of toxic Mercury amalgams in his eleven cavities, I would sing God's praises in the choir that I had read about in the church bulletin. It happened. My promise and the fact that I loved to sing Christmas carols, I made my way to Blessed Sacrament Parish in November of 2001 for the first choir practice of my life. Though I felt apprehensive, I couldn't stop myself from going into that church. It was as if I felt my soul pushing my body to go. A promise is a promise, at least in my book. I thank Jennifer that she and God work together. On my first or second choir practice, she stopped the whole choir and asked me if I could read notes. I thought I was in trouble, but instead she liked my voice. Months later, in February of the year 2002, she called and asked me if I'd be interested in becoming a cantor? Even though I didn't know what one was, she explained and I said, "Yes."

Looking back to my childhood, this is a dream of mine that I had always felt but had given up on coming true. Singing has always been a part of my life, it is just that no one noticed, but I secretly hoped they would. I can still see the picture in my head, me sitting on the bumper of our trailer in our driveway on 187 Mercer St., Chatham; Ontario.

I was not more than five or six years old. I am singing all of the song, "I Can't Smile Without You" to my grandma Elizabeth in heaven. She is my mother's mother, but she died when I was only seven months old.

Though unable to explain, I have always felt incredibly close to her. My mother attests to not speaking to me about her but she tells me having her baby girl helped her to get through her mother's death. She says before my birth, my grandmother had a dream that I would be a girl and she told my mother that she saw me when I was grown up.

I'll go back to singing. Only once, in an early grade, I was pulled aside by a teacher and told to move my lips, not to sing. I can still see a little girl named Lori-Ann standing there with me. Though I know that comment confused and hurt me, it did not change my love for singing. I still remember singing, "Angels We Have Heard On High," with my class at the Grade 2 Kiwanis Music Festival. I remember begging my best friend and cousin Janay to sing with me on her tape recorder. We were both born on Feb. 28th, me three years older, born in 1970. She was killed in a freak auto accident in 1992 while I was in nursing college. I still can see myself standing at the bookstore, my aunt, Janay's mother, standing behind me and asking me why I was buying a book by Elizabeth Kubler-Ross, "On Death and Dying." I heard about her in college, I told my aunt. This was 3 days before Janay's death. That was my dear Janay, God knows that I wouldn't sing solo in front of anyone else. I was a painfully shy little Catholic girl who loved the songs in the hymnal, though I sang about as loud as a church mouse. Church hymns, drawing and the challenge of academics were the only sustenance that got me through those dreaded school years. In Grade 5 it meant so much to me to choose a 'Holy' card for every perfect spelling test. I still have them. I learned about the 'Beatitudes' from Sister Rachel. In 2002 at World Youth Day, I was thrilled to hear Pope John Paul II talk about the importance of the 'Beatitudes.' At the top of my schooling list I remember the sense of honor that I had felt at being asked to crown the Virgin Mary in May of Grade 6; just as my mom had done in her day. Mind you, I still remember the sadness in my heart when someone that I considered a friend did not treat me well because I had been asked. I was shocked. I did not feel that school brought me much in the way of happiness. My biggest reality was trying to understand why people couldn't be happy for each other and thoughtful of one another's feelings. I'm still trying to understand that one; God loves us all.

I was a painfully shy, quiet girl who felt socially inadequate. The fact that my shyness was commented on frequently and in a negative tone, only made me feel I was a faulty human being. By the time high school rolled around, I despised myself. Thank goodness that I've turned that around too, with work and time. I thank my dad that he let me take the 'Dale Carnegie Course' at age 17 when I begged him. I also am thankful that he pushed me to get the job at 'McDonald's.' I also must offer thanks to my husband. At age 19 I met a kind and seemingly selfless young man who truly loved me. His kindness made me believe that I was something. I slowly began to give love to myself. In this same year I quit 'Western University' and came home after two months as I became extremely sick with 'Mononucleosis' and 'Strept throat' at the same time. It took me a year to recover.

But in that next year, at the age of 20, I took it upon myself to take singing lessons. I treasured the "Ave Maria" and "Panis Angelicus" that were taught to me by Christine Wilcosz-Thompson. I felt them deeply enough that I frequently sang them to my children while pregnant with them. I also thought it important that little Daniel, the fetus, should listen to 'Mozart' also. I particularly adored "Ave Maria." Now "Panis Angelicus" has resurfaced; though until 2002, I struggled with hitting the note high E. These songs were committed to my memory twelve years ago. At the present time I treasure them so deeply that I literally feel I might burst with joy, reverence and gratitude when I sing them.

But getting back to the year 2001, I would feel numbness in my hips, my knees and my thighs. A chiropractor couldn't explain it. I couldn't understand it. To add to the mystery, it had been two years that every time I went for a walk around a block, I would feel tingling move up my legs. It was a buzzing feeling like being plugged in. But never once did it strike me as a good energy buzz, like the energy that I feel when I'm the recipient of Therapeutic Touch. This I found disturbing. I did have disease oriented thoughts from time to time about why I would feel this, but I quickly put them to rest, trying to talk myself into the fact that it had to be good energy that I was feeling.

At this time my greatest frustration was my right hip going out of place. I felt like a broken marionette trying to walk. I went to a chiropractor for the first time in my life because I needed help. Dr. Lemak would often tell me that my hip was out a mile and put it back into place. My husband couldn't understand because he didn't know what it felt like to be me nor did he trust that what I was experiencing so frustrated and infuriated me. I only needed to be rid of the pain and discomfort and walk easily but all he could see was some imagined addiction because he couldn't trust me to know what I was doing? Would anyone like to go and waste their time and money at such places, if unneeded?

He acted like it was his body, if only it truly was his body, then he could feel what I was feeling. I don't think he ever imagined what it was like to be in my shoes. He certainly didn't try to, the time that I begged him not to remove his condom without telling me. I told him that I had a painful stomach ulcer and I was not ready to be pregnant again. Granted, I did open myself up to spirit, months before. You see; I realized that I'd been selfish in saying that I wanted children three years apart. At this time it hit me; it really wasn't up to me. I would accept whenever a little soul was ready to come to me because I knew that I had to be open to God's will and the will of the little soul.

CHAPTER 2
My Daughter Coming To Be

On Dec. 14th, 1996 I found out that my husband didn't listen to me. I felt violated again and I was angry. Angry, but I wanted to go to sleep. For me anger and sleep do not go together because I feel things too deeply. Neither did it help that my husband could once again sleep so easily when I was upset. I was ready to go downstairs and take one of my sleeping pills.

I feel that all of this is the reason that I was given the gift of what I will call a picture. A picture etched in our steam-condensed bedroom window. The window positioned beside me. I was taken aback. The meaning was clear. The clearing in the steam revealed the picture of an angel. It was the profile of an angel, about twelve inches high. The wing was big. Immediately next to and facing the angel was the profile of a tiny, little person.

I knew the angels were telling me that my husband's lack of listening would cause a second baby to come to me. God was letting me know what was going to happen and at the same time He prevented me from taking a sleeping pill. I calmed down instantly. Anyone who knows me; knows this isn't a usual occurrence when I'm extremely upset. I fell asleep immediately and peacefully. Exactly two days later, I felt the pain of ovulation. It was Sunday morning, Dec.16th, 1996. I was amazed that it was happening. That's when she began, our little girl, Samantha. She was born on September 10th, 1997, nine months later; exactly two years and one week after her brother.

Now as I sit here on Dec 10th, 2002, I recognize something when I look at the free flowing, no objectives, watercolor painting that I did yesterday at my monthly 'Waldorf parenting group.' I saw in my painting something that brought me back to the steam-condensed window message of Dec. 14th, 1996. I became aware that even though I had forgiven my husband, I had never thanked him for what he did. He had told me that those two times he had removed his protection or rather mine; he said that he had felt as if God wanted him to do it. Now I can look at the situation and realize its truth. So, I thanked him for the gift of our precious little daughter to share life with us and; our beloved son. I got pregnant with Daniel because of my desire to have a baby. I knew that I had just ovulated because of the pain. The purpose of their close births is further seen when I watch our two children interact with each other. They were meant to be that close to each other in age. They have been best of friends, which is such a blessing as we live out in the country. It does however, require incredible parenting skills, which I have learned is an ever changing and evolving art. Yes, making mistakes when you know you could do better, otherwise known as learning experiences. My children are my best teachers and friends, not to mention the fact that I think they could prepare me to work as a diplomat with the United Nations some day.

Amazing, both my children conceived within a day of each other; born a week and two years apart. This happened to the woman with irregular periods. I realize that this was a gift too, for I had never felt the pain of ovulation except for the two days that they were conceived.

This is one of the joys of being a highly-sensitive person. And even though all is forgiven, the coming of a beautiful child did not give excuse to my husband to keep disrespecting me by removing his protection frequently when he bloody-well felt like it. He promised that he would stop but never did! I couldn't believe it when my prominent gynecologist told me, when I brought it up, that he thought this the reason my menstrual cycle had stopped for a couple of years, out of my fear of becoming pregnant again. I believe it had a lot to do with self-preservation. The haemorrhaging that took place after the birth of my daughter; let's just say if it weren't for hospitals, I probably wouldn't be here. I was put on intravenous. Even though labor was very painful, it could not compare to the pain that I felt when the nurses kept pressing forcefully on my abdomen, massaging it vigorously to try to get the bleeding to stop. Only recently will I not grimace at the thought of it. Now I believe that both fear of becoming pregnant again and the poisonous effects of Mercury in my body played their joint roles in messing with my endocrine health. Now you may ask why I bring this up when I have forgave? Part of it is cleansing completely of hurts. The other part is the realization that the trust issue with my husband is not completely healed. It has only taken other avenues. Granted the roads weren't as treacherous, but they still led to my heart.

The issue of respect has grown into something that I demand. I deserve it. We all do. Is there some reason that some of us on this planet don't think we have to take responsibility for our behavior? We must take a good hard look at ourselves in order to grow. Yes, sometimes that hurts, but there is no need to beat oneself up, instead refuse to give up! KEEP TRYING. God knows we all have work to do, that's why we're here. BUT WHAT IS MOST IMPORTANT!! WAKE UP!! PEOPLE ARE WHAT MATTER!!!

I started taking 'JC Tonic,' a Chinese medicine that is a natural, herbal tonic in December of 2001. Over the course of a year, I now realize in January of 2003, that the tonic dug up the buried garbage that lay smouldering quite silently inside of me. It was not meant for the 'osteopenia,' the beginnings of osteoporosis that I was diagnosed with in the year 2000. But, that's part of the reason that I was so angry and fearful at not having a menstrual cycle. A woman needs the hormone 'Estrogen' to more easily form new bone. I didn't want to keep having the bones of a seventy or eighty year old woman at the age of thirty-one.

I remember Christmas time of 2001; I couldn't lift the children because my right hip was still going out of place. Only after, did I discover the psychosomatic meaning of hip difficulties in one's body. It stands for, if one looks into the studies of 'Louise Hay'—LACK OF SUPPORT. And isn't that ironic that the right side of the body is associated with our male issues, left side is female issues. My parents accompanied my two children and me to midnight mass because my husband said that it was too late. He said that he wanted to go to sleep because he didn't feel too well. The children so desperately both wanted to go with me to midnight mass that they were crying, screaming and telling me that they would not sleep, they would follow me. My parents saved me.

What started out as an emotionally tumultuous evening changed. It was Christmas Eve; the music we were singing upstairs in the choir loft was beautiful. My daughter was sleeping on the pew under the pipe organ, my son sleeping beside my parents on the pew downstairs. Because of all of this I had a deeply spiritual experience. I was so happy and had enormous appreciation for my parents, who because I was unable to, carried both my children out of church and then later into our home. So, even in the midst of turmoil, there is beauty. It even carried into Christmas Day. My daughter, who had been under the pipe organ, was sleeping peacefully until the closing song, "Joy to the World." When Marilyn started the organ, Samantha felt its resonance and vibrancy. She was startled such that her body shook, then quickly went back to sleep. Upon awakening Christmas morning, for the very first time, we heard our daughter singing, "Joy to the World."

I also remember the turmoil of the frequent vertigo that plagued me for nearly a month, beginning in December of 2001. I would walk into the kid's school and get so dizzy that I would have to stop and stand there, afraid that I would almost fall over if I didn't. I couldn't believe no one ever noticed or asked if I was okay; from where I'm at now, I look back and I'm not so surprised. Even as early as this, I remember kneeling down and having lack of ease getting back up.

CHAPTER 3

I Had A Dream

When January of 2002 came, I had a vivid dream, "I was a young boy and I was in a hospital. I was having great difficulty walking. My feet were turned outward. There were two doctors in front of me. I was holding something to keep my balance and my strength. I think it was an I.V. pole. I was TRUDGING, this I know. I still feel the dream though it is long gone. There is NO WAY I am going to give up. I see the path ahead of me. This boy didn't travel some short hallway in a hospital; he went outside into the world, going towards some other big building. I can see it still. He is trudging but he's not going to give up." This dream happened before the time my legs weren't working, as they should. It happened before the time that I put on my skates for the family skating trip, got on the ice, somehow got out to the middle and then realized the whole thing was a farce. I fell, landed on my lower back and knew I had to get off the ice somehow, if not, I was going to create a scene. I couldn't lift my legs to skate! As I now look back, I have tears in my eyes; the pain, the inability to use one's body, it's all too fresh. The fear I felt.

Oh God, get me through writing this! Though there are definite moments of joy interspersed with the painfulness of this year like our vacation to Barbados; which took place on my birthday and was a family kind of celebration of our 10th anniversary. I still remember having a relay race on the beach at the family 'Full Moon' party. People had encouraged me to run faster. I was trying but I knew I couldn't make my body do what I wanted it to do. I'm the reason that our team lost. The stairs at the hotel were always something too. I had to think about and gather my inner strength before going up. I guess that dream was supposed to happen. It somehow gave me comfort in its foreshadowing, that somehow all this was supposed to happen, that I shouldn't be alarmed. This is a good thing because stairs only became worse. It came to the point where I'd be at home and think, "Oh no, I have to go up the stairs, again." It took an incredible conscious effort, extra work that I didn't need. Running up the stairs was a physical impossibility and hilarity. In the months that followed, I tried different healing techniques. I even tried acupuncture, where the man implied it couldn't really hurt like I said it did. I informed him that I was highly sensitive. He soon came to realize that I could feel where and how the energy or 'chi' moved through my body.

Acupuncture wasn't long lived. I am an easy, loving, flexible person that deserves respect. I quit going to him because I was paying for a service and not being respected. Now I reiterate, I deserve respect at all times; whether paying for it or not, we all do. Maybe if I didn't give it, I wouldn't demand it. But ;I do give it. That's what love is all about! The symptoms at this time included my numb toes. I couldn't feel it when the acupuncturist had beat a little metal tipped hammer against it to encourage blood flow. I especially couldn't feel it in the left big toe.

At Dr. Frank Little's, a chiropractor recommended by my sister-in-law, I couldn't feel the sharp object that he ran across any of my left toes and portions of my foot. How I longed to feel some pain, just to know that 'feeling' might be coming back.

I went for massages for the first time in my life. I couldn't believe how painful they were. The sore spots on my body! I had never experienced such painful spots on my flesh! But somehow, even though the pain was tremendous, these spots needed to be rubbed and massaged to get relief. Most of these areas were in my legs and lower back. I was blessed because the woman who worked on me was a healer full of compassion; love and she let God's wisdom guide her from within. During this entire year, parts of my body were numb. There were times that my hips and genital area were numb. Only once was I numb above the midline of my body, my right thoracic side of course.

I remember 'Good Friday,' the numb feet, sitting in the choir loft, shaking them about, frustrated at them. My thoughts went back to the good fortune of having my daughter to sit there with me. It had only been weeks before that I had gone to choir practice without her and left her to my husband's care. Daniel was at home and my father-in-law was visiting too. I had had a hard day and told my husband that I desperately needed a break. Before I left, I distinctly remember asking the angels to keep watch over Samantha. As I sat in the choir loft that practice, I remember wondering how anyone could contact me if there was an emergency, but I quickly dispersed the thoughts because I thought myself thinking negatively. When I got home later that evening, I was in for a shock. I found out that our daughter had climbed thirty feet in the air to the top of our antenna because she was angry that I had left. She had even touched the shingles. My son told me this and I believed him instantly, my husband refused to believe that she had went this far, no matter what I said; until weeks later when his friend's wife had told him she'd seen what she'd thought was our little boy touching the shingles of our two-storey home. My husband had been in the garage with his dad and hadn't seen her climb and did not check on her when my son told him that she was climbing. This rocked my world; the trust issue again. That evening, when I was home from choir, I hugged her as I heard the story unfold. I was grateful to see her in her bed. I thanked God and the angels. Once the children were sleeping, I immediately went outside to sit by the antenna. I needed to look up and see where she'd been. I cried, I was angry but mostly grateful.

CHAPTER 4

Effects of Mercury Poisoning

When the 'Good Friday' service was over, our choir went downstairs. We followed in the line to the front of the church where people were genuflecting in front of the enormous wooden cross. All took their turn kneeling. As I stood in line, I was fearful that when I kneeled, I would either not be able to get back up or I would fall over. But I wanted to kneel. I did not want to give up. I knelt and was fortunate; I did get back up. It was a slow and labored process for me, but I somehow mustered enough strength, not that anyone could tell. Try to imagine how you'd feel if your legs were like this? That your muscles weren't working properly.

Take this summer for instance; when we'd take the boat to a swimming place, walking in the water became a daunting task. I was almost afraid that someone would notice but at the same time, it might have been nice if someone cared. I remember one instance when I wanted to go for a walk in the water to follow my son and my husband who were already quite a distance away. I couldn't walk more than five steps in waist deep water. I physically could not move my body any more than this. It was impossible. I sadly made my way back onto the boat, sat down and began to cry from the depths of my soul. How does one explain how horrible it is to be encased in a seemingly well-looking body that truly feels not?

I remember another time, weeks after that when I wanted to go with my family to see the geese on the little island. I wanted exercise too. I told my husband that I wouldn't make it if I couldn't hold onto him for balance and strength. So I did this, the whole time with my arm around his shoulders. When I let go and I did try a few times, testing myself, I couldn't make it. The muscles felt enamored with armor and I couldn't balance either. But since my husband couldn't feel what I felt, he didn't make too much of a deal out of it.

At least he held me up and as he told me, he was sick of telling me to go to the doctor. But I refused to go. And end up with some negativity laden disease sentence? "NO."

I am a registered nurse who graduated at the top of my class. I know what doctor's would say. But I believe in the innate healing capability of the body. How could I not? I nourish my body strictly and I have been doing so for a year. I am blood type O positive, I discovered this when I asked to have my blood tested for type. The learning of what to eat was courtesy of the "Eat Right for Your Blood Type Book I." My mom gave me this book. I consume only organic fruits and vegetables. The only grains that I'll eat are 'Ezekiel bread' which is based on a Bible recipe, 100% rye and I strictly cook with spelt flour. The meats and eggs I get are free range. The only time that I'd sway from this is when eating out; which is not often. It costs too much for the poor nutrition that one receives. I feel that in my body. I drink lots of purified water and that's all that I drink. No sugar; only what is in raw fruit.

Of course I made the exception for a weekly ice cream cone in the summer, birthdays and special occasions. I have been this strict and in my immune system, I feel incredible. It's funny that I started eliminating sugar completely because of the beginnings of osteoporosis. Sugar upsets the Calcium-phosphorus balance in the body. All year, I had been working profusely at rebuilding my bone mass. In June I was disappointed and greatly saddened to find that my bone density hadn't changed for the better, but also, it hadn't gotten worse. I felt it wasn't all about the big Calcium hype. My blood level of Calcium has been high, but there was some reason it wasn't getting to my bones. I knew there was a root cause to all of this. This kind of horror doesn't happen to people who take top notch care of their bodies and for the most part always have. My teenage years were full of aerobics and step classes. These are bone-building activities. You'll find in medical books that 'Osteoporosis' doesn't begin over night. Granted, having no menstrual cycle didn't help my bone building endeavors. This reminds me of another not-so-joyous time. I forced myself to do spin classes on stationary bikes and though difficult, I managed. I thought that I would be brave and try a step class. I had to leave the class after the on-ground warm-up because I physically couldn't lift my legs onto the short step. To do any sort of action would have been impossible. This wasn't humiliating, but discouraging. Well, actually heart ripping. Heart ripping comes when you tell your mother-in-law about this and she doesn't seem to care or truly believe you. Needless to say, I don't go to the gym anymore. I physically can't yet and truthfully I have discovered a lot better things to do anyway. None of them include a television; I despise it. For me, it is the biggest waste of time. I never turn it on. There are many better things for a brain and a body to do, like go for a walk down the street.

Luckily at the time that I write this, in early November, I can go for a walk and the worst thing that happens is that I get so dizzy, I feel like I'm going to fall over in the middle of the sidewalk, but I haven't. I do, however, have to sit down for fifteen minutes afterwards, usually in my car until my head stops feeling like it is rotating. I forced myself to walk, to build up my bones. There were times that it became a battle; soul and mind against body. I never gave up but the word trudging is a totally appropriate word, especially when your muscles are coated with metal. An inner suit of armor, upon the legs and of course using the heaviest metal you can find to give you the full effect of what I endured.

On the subject of metal, I went to a chiropractor who did a hair analysis; cut and sent it to a Toronto laboratory. What a coincidence, I had been wondering where you could get a hair analysis done? After he checked out my x-ray, which I requested to make sure that my back was okay which really it wasn't; my spine was twisted. I then looked up "Lordosis," which he said that I had. There were muscles visible on the x-ray that normally shouldn't show up and I found out that I have four lumbar vertebrae instead of five like most people. For me that wasn't the missing link and my major problem. My hair analysis results showed it. There was the presence of heavy metals. There was Mercury, Lead, Silver all in good amounts or rather bad amounts and Aluminum was very high. It's odd, the strong presence of Mercury and Silver; that's what was in most of my teeth. A not-so-nice touch is a root canal that turned my gum grey because it had corroded after being with me for only two years. I became a detective and felt great when I cracked the case of how incredibly young I was when I got my teeth filled with this poison.

"Oh, and don't worry," they say. "About the baby teeth you got filled, they are gone right?" they continue.

Never mind that you had to breathe in heavy metals when you were a child. What about all those vaccinations that contain Mercury and Aluminum? Of course being a nurse I had to get more. Now they are pushing everything on children too. Fear based society you know. Well, guess what? Some of us are bringing in the love, positive thinking, trusting and listening to our bodies along with the, 'you are the creator of your own destiny' attitude. This probably brings out the question, "Why isn't everyone so ill?" Well, I feel there are many ill people living under the shadow of a disease name when there are other attributable factors at work. If the only reason that I'm on this planet is to offer awareness to those who want to build a better world, so be it. It is correct to say that all do not hold onto the metals in their body, as strongly. Some bodies are better at disposing of them. I have learned a great deal. And because I am a R.N., I have access to buying and selling homeopathic remedies from a reputable company in Quebec whose products are manufactured in Germany. In their literature I have discovered that there are four different terrain typologies. In reading I have discovered that the category I meld with is 'Leutic,' the type that is prone to the deposition of toxic materials.

Did I mention that my previous dentist in town suggested that I might have Fibromyalgia and on the same day his hygienist offered that I might have M.S., I told her that you get the same symptoms from Mercury toxicity. The only hilarity I found in all of this is that even in the medical profession, it's seemingly impossible to have these two diseases at the same time, especially with pronounced severity within the course of one year. That and my heart knew different. This same dentist told me that he gets his blood level of Mercury checked every month and it is fine. I told him that different things affect people differently, that maybe he wasn't sensitive to it. If I could talk to him today, I'd tell him a different story. I would tell him that blood tests measure extracellularly; what's outside the cell, not intracellularly; what's inside the cell, such as a hair analysis will do. I'd recommend he do that to make sure it's not a problem for him.

CHAPTER 5

Divine Consolation

Many days in 2001 before I had the amalgams out, I found upon waking from bed that walking wasn't like it used to be. I'm pretty certain that I looked like a tin man trying to walk, a tin man with lead boots. Yes, this year has been a huge test of my inner strength. I think that I even started to spook the chiropractor so much with my symptoms that he suggested M.S. to me. This was before he gave me laser therapy with the electrical boost. The next day, I was totally numb from the waist down. I couldn't feel my behind on the toilet seat and I am dead serious. Ironically, we were at the movie theatre watching the movie "Signs." It was one I had wished to see, and the fact that our parish priest Fr. Jim Williams recommended it, it only enticed me further. I knew it was something that I had to see. In the movie, the actor recalled his wife's death. She was pinned to a tree by a truck; she couldn't feel anything from the waist down. As I watched the movie, I felt as if someone had walked upon my grave. It was almost otherworldly; the wife numb from the waist down on what was the day that I first experienced this symptom in myself. In the movie they kept her alive so that she could say good-bye to her husband, afterwards they pulled the truck away and she died. Ironically the man, a preacher, completely lost his faith in God over this.

The strange part is that I've never lost mine; in fact it was incredibly strengthened for me on Oct. 15th, 2002. That afternoon while the kids were at school, I finally took the time to sit down and rest instead of doing some kind of work. I was reading a book that touched on St. John of the Cross and the 'dark night of the soul' to which I was grateful he wrote about. I totally related to this. Then I read about a priest who did healing work. That's when it happened. In those moments nothing else existed. I thank God for that day and the message given with clairaudience to me. I had the absolute knowledge and feeling of a divine Fatherly presence. It began with a clairaudient instruction to immediately put my book down and lay my hands over my abdomen. I began to feel some energy. Then; I was told to be prepared to write down His words so that I would remember them exactly. Then with clairaudience I heard: "I love you, I will always love you; I will never be apart from you." After that, I felt the love. A love so great, it is like nothing I had ever humanly felt. This love was so great and so unconditional. I had no inhibition. I began to shout out loud to God, "I love You!" I couldn't stop telling Him how much I loved Him. I was trembling, crying tears of joy, and my arms were outstretched to heaven. Incredible is not even a good enough word to describe the love of the Father. Many times in the recent past, I had asked God what I was supposed to do with my life because there was so much that I loved to do. I never really expected an answer because I felt it was my job to figure that one out. But while all this happened, I felt knowledge imparted on me and it also came as a feeling over my stomach. It totally surprised me. This is the whole reason my gravitation toward Parish Nursing took on such fervor.

I was also made aware at the time that this happened that I would not get completely better until all of my Mercury amalgams were removed and the detoxification process was complete. When the mystical experience had settled, it was like I didn't know where time had gone. I was at peace and I was in awe of the incredible love that God has for all of His children. I had to keep telling Him how much I loved Him, still crying of course, even as I was in the bathroom. I kept repeating the words that I had heard with clairaudience as to not change or lose even a word. Then I collected myself and went upstairs to write it in my dream journal, the one with the angel picture on the front cover. Though this experience was by no means a dream, it was reality. As I was writing my experience down, I still couldn't stop crying. After I had the words down, I wanted to write the rest of the experience. I had to go downstairs and examine the book that I had been rereading. I was curious. I wanted to find the exact spot where I'd stopped reading. It was a blur of course, so I had to retrace my footsteps. When I did, I was surprised at where I'd been in the book. I didn't remember. That is not something I often say. Of course being me; I had to finish where I'd left off. I always seem to be the detective trying to connect stuff. After that day, my muscle coordination definitely improved. I could skip again! Previous to this, I was unable to skip. It had been a physical impossibility, no matter how fervent my efforts. I remember having a little hop in my step as I went up to the pulpit to practise the psalm with Marilyn. Sunday, two weeks later, I had the privilege of proclaiming the beautiful psalm, "I love you Lord, I love you Lord my strength." I could not wait to offer it to

God in church and every time that I practised it. I still have that one permanently implanted in my mind. Later in the week, I took pride in showing my parents how I could jaunt up the stairs. Just as I had shown my dad in previous weeks that I could not run up stairs, even though I looked perfectly fine. I guess I wanted someone to believe what I was going through. That time of course, prompted my dad to tell me to go to the physician so that I could at least get a diagnosis. I looked at my dad, smiled and said, "I am sorry to disappoint you dad, there's nothing wrong with me except for the fact that I'm full of heavy metals."

CHAPTER 6
The Poisoning Story Continues

But back to where I was, considering the fact that God is within each one of us; that would be the only way that I'd say I lost any faith in Him; because there were many times this year that I lost faith in certain people. ALONE would be a good word to sum up this year. It has been an incredible test of my strength. Perhaps, that's why the aforementioned experience happened to me. There's something about feeling understood that makes a huge difference in one's life. This is one thing that hearing my current priest's sermons has done for me this year, 2003. He has offered me comfort and support without knowing it. Quite a few times, he couldn't have done better if he'd read my mind; his sermons were in synchronicity with my feelings and perceptions. It has become obvious to me that God has ways of shining a light in the darkness, even if it's only for a moment. Did I mention that when I was numb from the waist down that I couldn't feel the temperature of the water in my bathtub? I had absolutely no idea how hot or cold it was, until the upper half of my body was immersed in it. And on this day, well actually the Saturday after that Friday movie, my husband was getting worried. I can realize now, but at the time it added incredible blackness to what was probably the darkest day of my 'dark night of the soul.' He suggested that I was ill because I ate so healthy, that I should in fact eat like normal people. He suggested that I should think positive, that my negative thinking and focus on my health problems was creating them. I could have screamed, I may have, I don't remember. What an emotional slap in the face. I totally believe in the power of positive thinking. I'm the girl, who says, "What you fear, you draw near." I'm the one who says; "Don't tell a child they're bad or difficult." I tell them, "Behavior can be bad; people aren't." If you put people down, you hurt people in the present and that negativity sticks with people into their future. You would have to be an incredibly strong soul or an insensitive one to not absorb the likes of such candor. Maybe there was a time in my life that I wasn't positive but that was many moons ago when I lived with a fear-based attitude, but anyone who truly KNOWS me now, would know that I am ultra-positive. Needless to say, after hearing what my husband had to say, I had to take off and attempt a long walk. The only down side of being highly sensitive would be the incredible pain that you feel in your heart when no one really knows who you are and what you're going through. Those nights when I felt so solidly numb and devoid of feeling, one would think sleep would come easily. To the contrary, it was the most difficult sleep that I've ever attempted because I could feel the nerves inside my body going completely bonkers. The sensations were tortuous. I tried to shake my legs to make it stop, but it wouldn't. After a couple of hours, I somehow got to sleep, I'm not sure how, but I'm grateful. Trying to explain the horrible ordeal, well let's say it is something beyond human conception to think such events could exist inside someone's body without physical evidence. Yes, alone again. I'm glad the hair analysis came up showing metals as I knew in my heart it had to. I thank You, God that it did.

The only sad part is that it didn't mean much to most people. Everyone is too engrossed in medical diagnosis. But the chiropractor, he believed it; he never made another mention of M.S. or going to the doctor. He felt I would be capable of chelating the metals by diet.

Speaking of a chiropractor, when I mentioned the laser, the electrical charge and the symptoms I had; about the numbness and the burning sensations in my back and legs, well, the next time they used just the light. That night and the next day, I felt like I had ice water running through the veins of my legs and my lower back. It was making me frozen, even with blankets layered on my legs. Believe me, I'm used to cold hands and feet with having idiopathic Raynaud's disease, which by the way I also plan to lose. My friend Wendy agreed with me and suggested that when the nerves are congested with metals, they are not going to conduct messages properly.

But a dentist in London told me too; Mercury affects the nerves, which in turn affect the muscles. That pretty well sums up this year, doesn't it believers?

I thank God for the dentist in London and his conscientious removal of my nine amalgams. In August, the yucky root canal was the first to go. On Nov. 14th he said that the gum tissue between the two teeth was beet red and the reason was because the metals in the two teeth were interacting, not in a good way i.e. electrolysis, more like a charged battery. He said we were on the right path.

I thank God for Wendy, her flower essences and her hyperthermia chamber; the wet sauna used for chelating metals through the skin. I'm glad she's in town because the point I was at, I would have gone to the doctor near London to chelate the metals intravenously, I would do whatever it took. I'm guessing you could figure that out about me by now.

CHAPTER 7

Singing, I Enjoy Working for God

A couple of months ago, I had a dream that I was running with my children. That made my day. I guess I didn't mention that I didn't have the ability to run at least easily or with any coordination, nor could I skip. It was physically impossible. But since Oct. 15th, 2002 I can skip. It's time for a humorous moment. It happened this summer, on the civic holiday weekend. They said we'd sing in our choir if about seven of us showed up, I think there were seven of us, including Samantha. My feet were totally numb inside, my husband said that he'd meet us there, but he didn't. Our choir songs included my all time favorites, one of which was, "Be Not Afraid." I thought since there was only a few of us, we had to be loud enough to make up for the whole choir. The fact that I was so physically and emotionally pained and my favorite songs, well, I sang my heart out and it felt great. The next week at the kid's school, one of the boy's fathers said that he saw me in the choir loft as he was at a baptism and he said, "You guys sounded good. Wow, you sure were belting it out." This still makes me laugh.

I thank God for Marilyn and that she asked me to cantor the psalms and the Gospel acclamation at the front of the church in 2003; that she asked me to help lead the children's choir. I am honored and love to sing God's teachings and praises at the front of the church, just as I'm honored to spend time, teach and hopefully help the precious children so full of love and openness. I think we all need to work at keeping them this way by showing them a good example so that they in turn will shine their lights. I remember now in Grade 6, the report card where one of my teachers said, "Pam is a good student, quiet etc., DON'T HIDE YOUR LIGHT UNDER A BUSHEL, PAM." At the time it was an insult; I wasn't doing a good job is how I took it. Now, I find the message hidden behind this comment in one of my favorite places of the Bible, "the Beatitudes." There is the part about, "The salt of the earth,' just as it was reiterated time and again by Pope John Paul II when we went to World Youth Day. This was a definite highlight this year, though I am still amazed that I trudged through that one O.K. too, walking was a big endeavor for me. Then there is the part about, "Not hiding your light under a bushel." It's amazing what you find in your life when you let go of the end results. Hold on for the beauty! And though I said I've lost faith in humanity at times, it's not total. People like Wendy, the London dentist, Jennifer, my children and my mom have been there for support. I suppose I'm a bit of a "Pollyanna," and you know what? I'm not going to do a thing about changing the idealist in me. I believe in all of us.

CHAPTER 8

M.D.'s, Dentists & Me

I got my last amalgam out on Nov. 22nd, 2002. I was fine until an hour after I got home at which time I became completely exhausted. The next day, my legs were stiff and I couldn't walk easily. My legs were heavy and more numb than they had been in a long time. I had a headache, which usually I am not prone to, except after getting the last few amalgams replaced. I had incredible abdominal pain. Then dead exhaustion came and dizziness. But wait, this time there's more; depression hitting me. It hit me to the point that I knew it was more than the hurt that I was feeling because my husband went to work again that Saturday morning when I told him I wasn't well. By Saturday night, my husband told me to go rest and I found myself in bed at 6:30pm. Me, the same person who for the last month and a half; had been waking up promptly at 5am, my body zinging with alertness. On the evening of November 23rd, I laid there in bed until sometime after 8pm at which time I fell asleep. But before this happened, my thoughts were abundant with grief. I had concluded that I didn't want to be a part of this earth experience anymore. I was stable. I knew I would not do anything to harm myself, I am aware of the repercussions; but at the same time I had never before had thoughts that the children would be okay without me. So, I lay in bed and simply begged God to take me home. I told Him that I couldn't do this anymore. All I held onto was the kindness that my gynecologist had shown me on the morning before my last dentist appointment. He had been interested in all the information I had about my hair analysis, especially the Aluminum toxicity linked with 'Premature Osteoporosis.' He hadn't seen anyone my age with the decline in bone density that I had. He looked amazed at the changes in my reproductive system and said that he felt I would be getting a period soon. He thanked me for healing myself and I answered by saying, "My pleasure." Being a R.N. gone into a natural realm, it felt so incredibly good to have such a prominent person in the medical field be interested in my research and believe me. He truly was the saving grace of my toxic weekend. Still holding onto this with the grief still in my heart, I meditated. What happened during my meditation is a blur now. This isn't usual for me either. After this I fell asleep. As I have become so aware of in my life, I once again was thankful to God for sleep. It is so healing, relieving our spirit and body to help us get through another day.

I awoke the next morning, Sunday, with my left knee twitching. Upon arising, I joyfully found out it was 6:45am. I had gotten up at 4am, but managed to get back to sleep this time. Talk about joyful appreciation! I guess exhaustion must have helped. When I arose, I was drawn to observe my hands. They were uncontrollably, lightly shaking. Even though I did not feel well, I told my husband that I would make it to church to cantor at the children's mass. It was the 23rd psalm and I knew I had to sing it. It would be what I felt was the only joy and help I could hold onto that day. I wanted to praise God. So, I had my detoxifying bath with Epsom salts and had my usual heavy metal healing homeopathy with an extra shot of 'Mercurius.' Then I took 'Glutathione' to aid in detoxifying. I knew today, instead of the usual raw vegetables before church, I had to do my best. I took the time to juice the organic fruits and vegetables. That's one thing that reading 'Daniel' in the Bible has done for me. Its given me the O.K. that what I've been living this year isn't so odd. Its given me company, that I'm not the only human on the pure foods quest. 'Daniel' writes that somehow eating purely helps one to more easily communicate with God. Upon reading this section of the Bible again, I particularly decided that I would only eat organic vegetables and water before singing at church. It makes it easier to get ready in the morning.

Upon arriving at church, I was light-headed and dizzy. I appreciated Jennifer asking me how I felt that morning. Even though she said I didn't have to go up, I knew I had to. I explained this as helpful to me if I did go up. I wanted to do it. But slightly before going up, I was feeling my illness and having my doubts because of the pain that I experienced. I prayed to God to help me get up there if He needed me to proclaim His word because I deeply desired to do it. I had the most beautiful feeling of peace singing the 23rd psalm, "The Lord is My Shepherd." I sang it joyfully, feeling it in my heart. I confidently and meditatively didn't have to look at the words in the hymnal because it was ingrained in me. I was so grateful, earlier that week Marilyn had suggested, because my kids grabbed me when coming down from the pulpit the previous Sunday that I could sit up front with the reader and rest until the gospel acclamation. Looking back, I knew my children had grabbed onto me for a reason that last Sunday. After singing God's praises, I felt amazingly better than I had before.

Later that morning, I was saddened. While we sat at breakfast, my husband got paged and was going to go to work again. I was grateful that my parents would watch our children so that I could go upstairs and sing at the noon mass too. The ladies' choir would be singing "Redeemer Lord," which I passionately loved. I went and it felt wonderful to sing that song before mass. But afterwards, I became aware that I was not well, so I listened to my body and sat down at times when others were standing and when I did stand, I had to hold onto the pew in front of me. I felt so ill that I asked Jennifer if it was totally wrong to get communion twice in one day. She explained to me that it was, under most circumstances, but that I could have Father pray over me or give me the 'Last Rights.' After this mass, I felt so ill that I actually walked bravely back into the church and was going to ask for the sacrament. Everyone was gone by then and I accepted that it wasn't going to happen for a reason. I'm glad because even though the rest of Sunday was soul gripping with its moments of sadness, especially on an emotional level, it had its glad moments too. And though not completely better Monday; I had come further along the path to healing. Only after all this had happened did I look up the symptoms of Mercury poisoning. All of which I had experienced, I found as symptoms. No exception was the back, abdominal pain and extreme tenderness I experienced on the Saturday. Yes, my weekend was described to a tee, right down to headaches, trembling hands and depression, the book even listed suicidal tendencies as a symptom of Mercury poisoning.

And yes, even though the London dentist is careful and has special equipment to do the job, when you are releasing the world's most toxic heavy metal, it is inevitable that some is going to get into your system. The high point of all of this was the confirmation that I was getting. Mercury had played the prime role in my disheartening physical status this year. I had no doubt about this. My legs had been so heavy and numb after the Mercury was liberated from my largest filling. And although I knew I was on the road to healing, that exacerbation gave me an incredible fright. Somehow, it helped me to remember the day that I was walking along in our kitchen, my mom was over, and I said, "I can't wait to get all the Mercury fillings out." I said this because there had been a number of cancellations and I was frustrated with my health and eager to get rid of the garbage. What happened after I said this? Well, I immediately hit the floor. I fell flat out from standing to lying there. I was as flat as a pancake. My mom had told me to be careful walking. I said that I didn't trip; I just fell out of nowhere, the split second after I uttered those words. I said it must have been a truth. It happened another time that day, at church. I don't know what I had said or what I was thinking but I hit the pavement flat out. Those were the only two times this year and in my life that this strange occurrence had ever happened to me. The only other time I fell, I had stepped on a sharp toy and hit the ground, more painfully than the aforementioned experiences, I might add.

Isn't it ironic that exactly one week after I got my last amalgam out, I get the first menstrual period that I have had on my own in one and a half years. I did have a very small period that was medication induced in June this year, but the gynecologist said that he wouldn't have me do that again since I told him the medication made me irate. And isn't it further ironic that my menstrual period became noticeable immediately after being intimate with my husband. This same day, Nov. 30th, I made two errors at the Mass that I was singing at. This was the first time that I had sung the entire mass by myself on the microphone. My voice cracked while I was singing, "Peace I leave," both times on the word peace. I realized that evening that it happened for a reason. I realized even though I told my husband that I had forgiven him for the prophylactic fast ones that he pulled, I needed to go a step further. The two times on the word "Peace," had signified for me, the two times that my husband removed his condom without telling me before my beautiful daughter was conceived. I had forgiven because we have the most incredible, wise, loving and beautiful daughter. But the times after when my husband continued to do the same thing, I realized, I hadn't completely forgiven him. I think I was letting blame rule me in such a way because he had broken my trust and my heart concluded that I wouldn't be able to trust him again. I was waiting for him to prove himself worthy to be trusted again. Every time he made a thoughtless error, I was wounded again. This was a big and ominous measuring stick for a person to be held against. Not to mention, it kept me hurting myself. I have forgiven now completely. After reading two pages on the night of Nov. 30th from "A Mystic Path to Cosmic Power;" I realize that he did not know how he was hurting me.

I realize that this helps me to let go of the past and hold out optimism and unconditional love for the future, realizing that I control none of it. Also, I realized that evening; the ability to laugh at myself is a necessary quality. Furthermore, I had to accept that I hadn't quite reformed the perfectionist in me as much as I thought I had. I knew I still beat myself up harder than anyone else could ever attempt to. Life is full of learning experiences. This is the beautiful reality. We need to accept ourselves; this is the key to growth and change.

This brings me to the other event that happened on Nov. 30th, 2002. I realized that the Andrew we had been praying for in the last few weeks was a boy we knew. It came to me, literally, like a small punch in the stomach. I came to the conclusion when I fully realized the name of his mother, Maureen. I hadn't clued in when I first read it in his obituary because I never knew Andrew's last name. I was stunned, saddened and later went upstairs to read in my dream journal. This is the dream journal to which I've contributed fewer dreams than I have fingers on my hands. One that had always bothered me; was the one where I dreamt of Maureen coming to me on Mar. 4th, 2001 and saying, "When are you going to bring Daniel over here?" I had always assumed it was about the 'Montessori school.' I had visited there a few times; ready to enroll Daniel because he had utter disdain, unhappiness and fear at John Uyen School. That is until later this year, October 2002, when Daniel proclaimed to me for the first time that he liked school and the main reason was his teacher. I can see the change in him; the ability to handle himself and be active in his life, I believe a good deal of this is attributable also to the 'Steiner' notable 'change of teeth.' When the child loses his first primary teeth, it foreshadows a readiness for school. This comes from a Waldorf school perspective. Our Daniel lost his teeth later than average, his first one gone this summer. Daniel has had his tests of strength. I attribute this first hand because I sometimes receive the fall-out of his pained feelings. I can't say that I was any different as a child. But, he's handling things much better than his mother could ever have dreamed of as a child. I believe we are helping each other to grow.

The really strange irony is that Andrew had just come to Fatima. I have concluded that this seemingly obvious dream somehow didn't hold the meaning it appeared to. I realized this as I read the words I had written. There was no mention of a school name in my dream. Funny, somehow this year both Daniel and Andrew did end up at the same school. Daniel was there because French Immersion had split into two schools. Andrew was there because his parents moved him there. Over the last year or two, Andrew was the one boy that I held in my heart as someone Daniel would have at the 'Montessori school' if we made the transition. They had been the only two boys at their 'Kindermusik' session. They were both four years old and they got along well. This dream showed me that things are not always as they seem. The day that I found out about Andrew's passing, I looked over Daniel's photo album. In it I found a 'Kindermusik' photo with the whole group together and I also found a single one with only Andrew and Miss Noelle, their teacher. My children weren't even in it. Needless to say, I felt the pull to give this picture to

Andrew's parents. He looked so happy and adorable; I knew it belonged to them. Thus, I passed it to them in a card at the funeral home. In retrospect I only hope my timing wasn't bad, I thought they would like to see him so happy in his life.

Beneath this paragraph in my scant dream journal, I reread a dream that I had a few days after the 'Maureen' dream. It was about me auditioning as a singer. I was able to hit high notes that I hadn't hit before! I got the job and there's more peculiarity after that. This dream came the winter before I even joined my first choir.

On Sunday, Dec. 1st, 2003 since I knew that Marilyn was going to give me the opportunity to practice, "Panis Angelicus" on Tuesday Dec. 3rd, I figured that I must practice at home too. On this Sunday afternoon I taught myself to sing the high notes, the high E to be exact. I practised, "Panis Angelicus" at least seventy times that day. Plain and simple, I literally could not stop. I attained something I didn't think possible, but yet I believed and was determined.

I had a fun practice with Marilyn after Andrew's sad funeral. And even after that sadness, a kind lady told me I did a wonderful job on Saturday and that others had remarked that same comment. This was the evening that I messed up! I felt bathed in love. Another morning at the grocery store, a lady working the meat counter, Barbara, told me that she thought I had a beautiful voice and that she missed me last Sunday. She said I sang with vibrancy, she told me it gave her chills. This made my day. Truly this is my biggest dream and only purpose in singing is to praise God and touch people through scripture and song with the knowledge and feeling of His love for them. I am honored to even make an attempt.

CHAPTER 9

Christmas Time

With this in mind, I continued the journey on Dec. 24th, Christmas Eve. It was fun bringing Daniel to church to be a shepherd in the church Christmas pageant. What was not fun was being in the meeting room and once again being completely aware that stability and balance were issues. People standing too close to me, bumping into me or pushing me, made me feel like I was going to fall over. It further disheartened me, walking across the room and accidentally kicking a chair, which made me half trip. But at least for this beautiful mass, I made it down the aisle.

At my parents house I had a good time. When alone, I got the courage to ask my brother what he thought about the summary of our family's 2001 letter that I'd written and sent along with the Christmas card. He looked at me and said; "It was interesting." I was surprised. I wrote that it was the hardest year of my life and that's all he had to say. I sat there at the dinner table mulling this over in my head; my brother sitting beside me. I picked up a walnut and the nutcracker. I began to crack it and then the nut mysteriously slipped out. I shot my brother with a walnut. He looked stunned. I laughed, my heart managed to get its feelings out somehow. Alan showed me how to properly use the nutcracker i.e. with the nut facing down. Though I felt sad, I somehow, for the first year ever diplomatically got the children and Alan to agree to open their presents, one person at a time while the others watched. I still felt sad. I sure was glad to drive to church by myself as I had the need to cry a little before midnight mass. I managed to get a few tears out. What I was not prepared for, was walking down the aisle for the candlelight ceremony. Though my feet no longer feel like beanbags, my legs at this moment felt like two-by-fours. I was looking forward to singing, "O Come, O Come Emmanuel" with the teenage girls; I wasn't going to give it up. But, neither could I believe what difficulty I would have walking and how obvious it was. I hoped that Father wouldn't think I was intoxicated. When I got up to the choir loft again, let's just say I was glad that I could sing so that I might release what I had just been through, mind you this is more emotionally reeking havoc on me than physically. But only two days prior to Christmas Eve, I had asked God again, "Why has my complete healing not come about yet?" This time, I became aware of the answer. I had realized that I had not fully been committed to living this experience here on earth; I believe I never had. When the going got rough, my head was in the clouds, not wanting to be here, shunning the fact that I had ever been placed on earth. I realized at this moment that I had come here for a reason and that I needed to be thankful and enjoy it. I needed to stop asking God to take me home when the going got incredibly unbearable. At this moment I made the commitment to God that I would not ask Him to bring me home until it was my time. I would strongly endure this place, it is meant to be and furthermore that God knows when my time to come home is, when my journey is done, and I trust that. I feel this Christmas Eve was my chance to honor the promise that I had made to God. I did not ask Him to free me from this place; I trusted and endured.

And believe me, it was not easy considering the test of fearfulness and loneliness this year has caused me to endure. But I will tell you one thing, I continued to aspire to health. I made myself dance to ABBA on Christmas morning when my legs did not want to nor did they make it easy, but this didn't stop me.

As we drove out to the Bay and got just beyond my mother-in-law's house, I felt a feeling of nausea and illness come over me. It hit me like a tonne of bricks. It was freezing cold outside but I desperately pleaded with my husband to open the truck window because I needed fresh air badly. Anyone who knows me; knows I hate the cold. Right away, I knew this peculiar because my immune system had not been bothered by even a cold for the last year. This is complete honesty, believe me, I know and appreciate good health; I was the little girl who got sick so often throughout my life. I felt completely better within about three minutes. How peculiar though? When we finished my husband's traditional 'making sure the water is still in the lake' escapade and returned to my mother-in-law's house, I went to hug his grandma and discovered that she and her husband were sick. They wouldn't even shake hands because they kindly didn't want to pass it to anyone. It sounds weird, no doubt, but for me it was freaky and reassuring. I'd have trouble believing it myself if I hadn't felt it in my body first hand. Somehow I was able to perceive things beyond myself. I have heard others who do healing work speak of this but I had never felt anything with this much strength before this Christmas Day. And no, I did not get sick later; what I felt was not mine. Believe me, I have had enough of my own to feel but it has nothing to do with my immune system. You should have seen me try to hide the fact that my walking abilities were not that of your average human being. But I am still a nurse, knowing our grandparents were sick, I made certain to avoid any sweets that would depress my immunity. I wasn't the least bit tempted by them anyhow. That's not me anymore. I could care less about that kind of stuff.

And guess what? Christmas Day turned out to be the best one ever! This was a dream come true. My mother-in-law asked me to sing, "Amazing Grace" while my son Daniel played it on the piano, since she was going to miss Daniel's performance on "First Night," the Chatham New Year's Eve celebration. I did all five verses by heart. My mother-in-law asked me to tell her about the Divine experience I had on Oct. 15th, 2002. After, that is, I mentioned I had had an experience, which I would not have mentioned if it hadn't been for the little religious book she had gotten me for Christmas. We talked in the kitchen. She believed me! She said that she had something similar, but different, happen to her. She understood how others might feel about it and I told her that was why I had mentioned it to few people. She told me that she told everyone she knew about her experience when her father died and she thanked me for sharing. She asked if we could talk more about it sometime. Later, I asked Linda what her favorite Christmas Carol was and she said, "O Holy Night." Oh, was I excited because that was my favorite too. We decided to sing it. I was so happy. The lady's choir had not sung it on Christmas Eve and I had totally longed for it. I felt completely fulfilled to sing it now with my mother-in-law. Then my husband suggested that I sing, "Panis Angelicus." I was shocked and thankful. His family agreed and I sang it, my daughter joining me with a mock presentation in the background.

When it was time to leave, my young brother-in-law thanked me for singing, complimented me on my voice and said that I hit every note perfectly. My other brother-in-law thanked me later too. I was the recipient of hugs and much love that evening and I was happy because I received the singing Christmas that I had always dreamed of.

We listened to ABBA on the way home again. I love the song, "I Had a Dream." It couldn't describe me better if I had written it myself. "I had a dream, a song to sing; to help me cope with anything. If you see the wonder of a fairy tale; you can take the future, even if you fail. I believe in angels. Something good in everything I see. I believe in angels when I know the time is right for me. I cross the street, I have a dream. I have a dream, a fantasy; to help me through reality. And my destination; makes it worth the while. Pushing through the darkness; still another mile. I believe in angels. Something good in every thing I see. I believe in angels, knowing when the time is right for me. I cross the street; I have a dream."

But my story gets better. Before I left my children's bedside that 25th day of December after reading the Christmas meditation about the story of Jesus; I did Therapeutic Touch and Jin-Shin Jyutsu on them. I left my sleepy daughter's room and went to lay with my son and give him his turn. Within minutes, I felt a wave of energy begin to enter me. It was making me tremble and shake and I knew healing work was being Divinely imparted on me too. I got tears in my eyes, smiled, chuckled and thanked God, thanked Jesus, the Holy Spirit and Mother Mary. I could barely speak but asked my son what he was feeling. He said that he could feel the energy going into him and the color that he saw was white. After this experience and I kissed Daniel good night, I for some reason could hardly wait to get up and walk. Walking felt easy, I got brave and I thought I would check out my dancing ability too. Even though I forced myself and I mean forced, truly you'd have to live in my body to know what I mean. I danced to ABBA music in the morning; but it was different now. I felt normal. It was easy. I was so happy! I got up to our bedroom and danced and danced. My husband said that I was setting myself up for a fall. I told him to not give me that negativity; I could dance because my legs worked and I was darn well going to love, appreciate it and enjoy every moment. I am certain that he later understood the difference in me. I think the 'silly goose;' smiling and laughing so much that it probably looked as if I'd burst, did it. My behavior probably convinced him. I told him what had happened when I worked on Daniel. Later, still in our bedroom, as Scott read a video cam manual, I practised my singing for the Saturday, Dec. 28th church service. I sang everything, even "Panis Angelicus," of course. I was in a total state of bliss. Merry Christmas!!!

Christmas 2003, I went to church by myself because Scott and the kids made every excuse not to go. Scott had left my car on empty and I could only give a $2.00 donation at church because I could only withdraw $20.00 from the bank machine. This was the maximum amount that would come out at the time and I had to save it for gas. After mass, I think that I shocked Fr. Joseph's "Christmas Day" because I asked him how one gets an annulment? He told me that one needs a divorce first. Live and learn.

CHAPTER 10

Concussion

I went down the basement to sleep because I couldn't sleep in our room. I missed a stair and slammed the left side of my head against the wall. I then fell hard onto my right side. All I could think was to thank God that it hadn't been a worse fall. At least I should sleep easily now. I gave myself a concussion. And do you know what? I had been right on both counts. For about three weeks, I found myself incredibly tired. A few times, I would fall asleep on the healing bed during the day because I simply could not go on. This is not Pamela; she simply does not have the ability to nap. I wish! That is, unless I give myself a concussion. Let me tell you though, I appreciated sleeping in past 6am, not to mention past 4:30am or 5am. That was what autumn consisted of for me. I would simply awaken at these times. It was always so sudden that when I would awaken, it was almost as if someone had shaken me and told me to get up, but of course no one had. I wouldn't even give in to meditating this early. I didn't want my soul to be rewarded for waking my body up insanely early and get in a habit. But fall two times; another time was after the Santa Claus parade. I fell when forcing myself to run a race with Daniel. He suddenly crossed in front of me and I lost my balance. Boom! I landed on the pavement. I didn't hit my head but I felt my brain get jarred. When you spend the late autumn season shaking your brain, believe me, by the time winter is here; it truly does become the season of respite. When falling down the basement stair, I knocked my hip out of proper position, as well as doing some serious damage to my head. But at least I got another chance to go to a chiropractor to talk about the damage heavy metals cause to people. He informed me that the damage can be permanent if not disposed of soon enough. I'm glad my garbage got brought to the surface when it did, so I can deal with it and have a positive outcome, God willing. He talked to me about seeing children who had been diagnosed with ADD. Their parents brought them. He recommended that their hair be analyzed and most often the result was high Aluminum levels. He felt these children had more positive outcomes the sooner that the issue was addressed. That reminds me, today I found in some papers that I had stored away, about metal detoxification that a chiropractor had given me in the summer. Mercury is said to cause an increase in Aluminum toxicity. Ding! Ding! Ding! We have a winner, or rather a loser. This makes me sad yes, but yet I'm happy. Following Christmas, I was thrilled at the opportunity to solo for church three times. The degree of happiness that I feel singing religious songs, praising God and the holy family and the angels; to put it simply, I can remember every event in my life that ever attained this level of bliss.

CHAPTER 11

New Year

I made an offer to Marilyn that I could sing "Ave Maria" on New Year's Day at 9am when I found out it was the Feast Day of the Blessed Virgin Mary. I have known and loved "Ave Maria" for twelve years. I sang it to my babies when pregnant with them and beyond. At first Marilyn digressed, I let it go knowing that my inner self had only to offer. But she called back an hour or so later, and it's really funny, I had the feeling it was her. She said if I was comfortable with it that I could sing it. I said, "Yes." I was excited but a little afraid; after all, we had New Year's Eve set up for Daniel to enjoy his first paying job as a pianist. His five-year-old sister was to accompany him on violin. I was M.C. and the vocal accompaniment for "Amazing Grace." Our family enjoyed ourselves tremendously. But walking in Tecumseh Park for the 9pm children's New Year's count down; was physically not a walk in the park for me. We got home at 11pm and I fell asleep easy. This is post concussion and spiritual courtesy I'm sure. I awoke with perfect timing for the 9am mass and "Ave Maria." I hadn't sung a solo of "Ave Maria" in public since my first and last Kiwanis Music Festival in 1990. It felt wonderful to honor Mother Mary on her Feast Day. One of the other songs, "Hail Holy Queen Enthroned Above," I remember singing as a young school child. It was so long ago that the words had changed from, "Sing with us 'Ye Seraphim' to 'You Seraphim." I had checked with Marilyn weeks earlier because I was concerned that I might accidentally forget and sing the old version. She said that would be perfectly fine, so I opted to sing the traditional version and enjoyed myself tremendously.

It was a wonderful New Year's Day. I was hopeful for the future. This was Wednesday and my last solo was to be Sunday. My daughter awoke and said she had a dream that she wanted to tell me in private. Since we had to be at church for 9am, we didn't have time for the private moment. I enjoyed singing at mass so much. My body's cooperation, well it didn't happen. The legs weren't heavy but they weren't moving steadily or balanced, it can't even be described with words. This was the first time that I had ever thought, let alone said out loud, "I don't think I'll ever get better." I told this to my mom as she watched me with full effort coming down the stairs from the choir loft. This was so unlike me to think or say. I felt really bad, really down and dejected.

But, I had my moments to hold onto. Like night time that New Year's Day when my daughter finally got the private moment with me to tell me about her dream. Samantha reminded me that she hadn't told me the dream yet. I asked her what it was about. She told me she saw Mother Mary in her dream and she was with an angel. They were across a fence. It was beautiful. Isn't it ironic that this same child desperately wants to join the Rosary Club even though that would make her the youngest one ever? Needless to say, I advocated for her. She was excited beyond words and also very eager because I was there.

CHAPTER 12

Bath Time

There was a night, while sitting in the bath and talking to my husband that I released some of my pain and burdens by speaking them. I wondered aloud if I was weird or off the beaten path to be living my life so strangely by most people's standards? I don't eat sugar and I despise television so much that I can't stand to hear it on. You know some of the rest by now. Immediately after I completed venting my despair, my questions about my life that usually I felt no doubt about, then something happened. The newly dried, fresh towels that I had hung there an hour ago, untouched and hanging perfectly; one of them just fell off the rack, plop! It might mean little to some people, but the painful emotional and physical state that I was in; it was all the answer that I needed to tell me that I was not alone living in such a manner. It's almost as if I was given support. I needed that. It lightened me right up.

My husband even looked perplexed when the towel fell. It reminded me of when I was in labor with my daughter, Samantha. The nurse had done an unpleasant digital check on me and told me that I wasn't dilated at all. I had waited for twelve hours of what I knew was labor before going to Victoria Hospital in London. My doctor had told me that I was dilated one centimetre, a week before I saw this nurse. I had even gone to the shopping mall to walk before going to the hospital because I wanted this labor to progress as much as possible naturally. After you have a 57 hour labor with your first child and get sent home because a different doctor tells you that you are not in labor, and the labor pains never stop and the next day you have to go back to the hospital; well, you don't want that to happen again, so you do everything in your power to make sure that they can't do that to you again. But guess what? It does happen again. The nurse tells me to go for a walk down the hall, and then she'll check me again and if she finds nothing, she'll send me back home to

Chatham. I walked down the hall crying and complaining. "What's the problem," my husband says. I could've wrung his neck. I feel desolate. I get back to the room thinking that I physically cannot endure another 57 hour labor. I get onto the bed and I sit there. In my head, I silently pray and ask, "Angels aren't you here with me?" It is a split second after I think this that something loudly falls off the back wall behind the bed and hits the floor. I turn to see and it looks like a stethoscope that was hanging on the wall. I smile in my moment of utter turmoil and hopelessness; the angels had let me know that I wasn't alone. Just after the nurse walked in to check me again, I explain to her again what the doctor had told me a week ago. She examines me. To me it is painful and harsh. Then she looks at me and says; "You have a dilation of three centimetres. I guess I just have short fingers." I guessed she did too. Thank you God for angels!

Basically most of the effects of my minor head injury have been put to rest. I can walk without being a dizzy duck. But there was still so much physical oddity going on. I can't walk easily. I thought it was because I hadn't done chelation in the sauna for a few weeks. Needless to say, I booked it and took my daughter with me. Supper was all ready on the go; chili was in the crock-pot. Today was the day that the 'Padre Pio' bread recipe Marilyn had passed onto me, would be ready to make and pass on to others. I thought O.K., I can detoxify. Now the impression I get from some people is that they think sauna and they feel it is something very nice. A relax, walk-in-the-park kind of thing. Ha! I find most of the time it's a test of strength, cook your body and pull the metal out, kind of endurance test. Usually I can make myself handle 20 minutes. Today, I hear with clairaudience that it is time to get out. After a couple of minutes I get out, I am very hot. I open the door. I can barely stand; I quickly grab a towel and boom. I'm down on the floor. I have my towel sort of on me. I am trying to sit up. I'm forcing myself to try and sit up on the floor but it's like I am being pushed down. Now my back is on the floor, I'm lying there. I'm getting frustrated. I need to fight this, get off the wooden floor and get dressed. I try to sit up again. I struggle almost like it is against some invisible force. I am determined. I sit up almost but it's like I get pushed back down. It's freaky. In retrospect, it's almost like an invisible person is pushing me back. I fling backwards. This time, I'm thinking that I can't lay here unclothed with a towel barely on me. I need to get dressed. I ask my angels for help. I get sitting. I somehow stand for a moment. I make it to the chair. Getting dressed is a huge chore. I feel like a "Weeble" wobbling. I am certain that I must also look like one. I get dressed. I make it to the door for a second, open it and call to my daughter to get our friend Wendy. I tell her how I feel. I manage to get to the healing bed, she says because my body somehow knows it needs it. She's right. She does "Reflexology" on me and it is incredibly painful in certain spots, especially around my anklebone. This is enough that it makes my foot jerk uncontrollably and it hurts. I am glad my daughter climbs up on the table so that I can hold her to get me through the pain. Wendy tells me the congestion; according to Chinese medicine is in the spleen channel. Of the symptoms she reads, most are mine, especially the leg weakness and the lack of bone density. My feet were jerking uncontrollably with pressure applied to certain points. This happening makes total sense. At home I was beginning to wonder why my feet were twitching, only over the last few days. The body has a knowledge all its own. Well, I feel good enough afterward to walk as normal as possible for me that is.

When I get home, I'm tired. I realize that I am allowed to take time for myself and stop working. I feel inclined to pick up my new, old favorite book that I had ordered about five years ago, "An Inquiry into the Existence of Guardian Angels" by Pierre Jovanovic. I read about three-quarters of it at that time. I find the part about the Saints and Stigmatics. At the time it is a little too deep for me. Not so now, I can't read enough of it. So I open my book, as I so often do, in doing so trusting that where I open to is where I need to read. What do I turn to? It is the page with the title "Padre Pio." This was the bread that I had passed to me in honor of him. Today was the tenth day, the day I was to cook it. Needless to say, I was flabbergasted and couldn't wait to read. I was amazed. This man was a priest who saw angels and talked to them, knew people's lives intimately without ever having met them, spent a good deal of his life with the marks of Christ on his hands and feet. He had been loved by people, but mostly treated poorly and despicably by his colleagues. When he died, the stigmatic wounds vanished, his body incorruptible. I was glad to know somewhat intimately the life of another saint. And my children, my husband and I; we enjoyed the bread. It was supposed to be a bread of 'Good Luck,' believe me, I would not refuse that; even though I tell my children that you make your own luck in life. I believe there is no good or bad luck. My son could not get enough of the "Padre Pio" bread. He couldn't help but complain that you are only supposed to make it once in your life, so he consumed all he could. We had fun. I was wishing to go to church that evening after Daniel's piano lesson; particularly because it was the Feast Day of Blessed Andre Bessett, a saint whose story had touched me deeply in years past. Alas, it was not meant to be, there was no service, even though Daniel had wanted to go with me after piano lessons. Instead, he spied a massive, mountainess snow pile in the church parking lot, accumulated by a snow plow's efforts of course. I walked over to the pile with him and he begged me to come up. Of course I said, "No, I can't." I had fallen and hit my head too much lately. Only minutes later I knew I needed to add some spontaneous fun, also there is no way I'm giving up. I was going to enjoy myself with my son. I cautiously and crazily went up. Happily I made it. I had cautious fun and talked with my son. Upon going down the snow mound, I prayed that I would make it safely. I did, mind you, need to go down on my behind somewhat.

CHAPTER 13

Park Trip

As I write this, I'm reminded of this summer at Rock Glen; a fossil hunting wonderland. I guess my insanity of testing my body reminded me of what I had forgotten this summer. I was brave this summer, but once again, I wasn't giving in. I climbed on huge rocks over trickling water. The whole time I knew that I was not being logical. I got some fossils and a big bruise on my hip, but I made it. I had fun with my family. Before we barbecued our supper, we wanted to go to the museum that lay at the top of the steep hill path. Looking at it, I knew it was giving me ominous forebodings, but I went anyway. I made it, well to the top anyway, going down was a different story. Somehow or other my foot slipped backwards under my ankle again. I say again because I had a less severe version on the stairs at home. I'm down; I'm hurt. At this moment I don't even think I can get down the hill by myself because my ankle hurts so badly. My husband doesn't seem to be worried or concerned for that matter. I'm not sure how, but I made it back down by myself. I went straight to the picnic table and began to profusely do Therapeutic Touch on myself. Later I put on some ice. I hobble over to the giant teeter-totter to watch the kids and make sure they are safe. My ankle hurts incredibly but it's not broken. At least a nice man who saw me fall asked me if I was okay. The next morning when I awaken, the ankle hurts tremendously but I am surprised there is not a touch of bruising or swelling. Not much good if you want your husband to believe you are in a lot of pain. But I made it through. The next day, my ankle doesn't hurt at all. The large purple bruise on my right hip however, I still had as a souvenir to remember our family trip by for a few more weeks.

CHAPTER 14

"Panis Angelicus"

Somehow, I manage to derive optimism. I went to church this past Sunday, Jan. 12th and enjoyed singing in the congregation. My husband told me I was kind of loud, that's why he didn't sing. This made me laugh. If I was loud, I didn't realize. I love to adore, respect and proclaim God's glory. I was thankful because we had been asked to bring the gifts up to the front of the church while Father Jim was there. When I heard this, I was on my knees praying that somehow Jesus would give me strength to walk without looking like I was severely intoxicated. The reason I was thankful was that the gift bearing was called off because the family who was having their child baptized would be doing it. At the same time I felt despondent because I figured that Jesus must have figured I really couldn't do it. Now I understand different, but at the time of mass, my lack of vibrant health, once again found me deep in prayer. So much in fact, there were times I found myself with tears in my eyes during the service. When the time came to speak, "Lord I am not worthy to receive You; but only say the word and I shall be healed." I resigned myself completely to the will of Jesus. Seconds later, in my head I clairaudiently hear, "It is over." I was surprised. I had deep reverence when going for communion. A reverence, which developed intensely for me since my research into the exact meaning of the Latin words in "Panis Angelicus." I researched it sometime in November 2003. I wasn't satisfied with the Internet site's translation. I looked up the song word by word. The Internet translation had said the part about "Pauper, pauper, servus et humilis," meant that the bread of Christ was for anyone, even the poor and humble servant. To me it never resonated because when singing this song, there is such a deep felt passion and forte during these particular words. I think, "Of course the bread of Christ is for everyone. Yes, the poor and humble servant, why wouldn't it be? If anything, I felt these servants would be most deserving, not an afterthought." Then as I was standing in my kitchen that morning, it hit me, literally but gently. That stomach area again. A poor man, a poor man, a servant and humble. I knew what the sentence really meant. It was a description of Jesus Christ. I shouted out loud, "It's about Jesus, it's about Jesus! "That is the reason this section of the song written by Cesar Franc exhibits such passion and vibrancy. It made sense to me now. I figured it out; with spiritual help I am sure. My interpretation of the whole song translates as: "Panis angelicus-Angelic bread; fit panis hominum-bread made for man; dat panis coelicus-bread dedicated to heaven; figuris terminum-the boundary of all beauty; o res mirabilis-oh miraculous event; manducat Dominum-eat of God; pauper, pauper-a poor man, a poor man; cervus et humilis-the most humble servant."

It now makes sense to me. I figured it out; with help I am sure. Excitedly, I began to sing the song. I walked over to our family room window and looked out while I was singing. The clouds were quite thick that day. For a confirmation that means something only to me, when I looked at the clouds in the sky, I saw a shape made by the small area of blue sky that they surrounded. It was not perfectly symmetrical but it spoke to me, I saw a star. I often stare at the clouds because of the sheer beauty, but this was different. I ran for my camera to get a picture. But if I had listened to my inner voice, I would have stared at the star a little longer because I knew it would be gone when I got back with the camera. It was. I have such passion for the song. I did from the moment that Sunday that I taught myself to hit the high notes that I had never attained before. I could not stop practising. I sang it at least seventy times. Now with me knowing inside what I figured the song to mean, I was on fire. It was about Jesus Christ and what He did for us; and the example He set for us. I deeply wanted to sing it at mass. On Dec. 28th, I would have that chance. Marilyn felt that the Saturday night mass would be the only appropriate one for me to solo this at. I got to sing it before mass, the day after I gave myself the mild concussion. Nothing could stop me. I was so happy; I wanted to praise Jesus. I felt a thankfulness and closeness develop toward Christ that was new to my life. When I sing it, all I want to do is look at the tabernacle. This is new for me. Even as a child, it had always been God the Father that I had called to in my heart. And since my experience on Oct. 15th, 2002, I have been prompted to want to know Christ further. I had always feared Him, but that was changing. I asked and I received. I simply want to sing praises to Jesus. He came to earth, gave Himself by enduring incredible pain and by the example of His life gave us the perfect example of how we should live with one another. Marilyn allowed me to quench that thirst. I was thrilled to bring this song to people with the passion that I felt for Jesus, hopefully passing it on. This is the reason that I wish to share.

CHAPTER 15

Chiropractic Visit

It's January of 2003. Brrrr! Since I had given myself the mild concussion, I had also begun to put my hip out again when I fell. I got an appointment with Dr. Lemak because I had known it was out. I had gone to a different chiropractor; he didn't get it in place. Dr. Lemak was always great at putting the hip back in when he said it was 'out a mile.' Once again, I am so thankful to my mom. She knew how I felt and told me she was driving the kids and we had time to get a few needed groceries before, so we stopped in the big Zehrs. Thank you God, my mom took me. I could barely walk. I wouldn't have made it through if it weren't for her help and the grocery cart to hold onto. You know it's bad when Pamela accepts help from the cashier to lift the groceries into the cart. The chiropractor, Dr. Lemak was great. He told me that I was so dizzy and fatigued because I had gotten a concussion. He had put my hip beautifully into place, but the next morning it was out again. Later, I was told that sleeping on the couch in the basement had probably caused this.

In all actuality I knew better, but somehow when I'm extremely angry at my husband because of his choice of words, or rather his speaking without thinking and his behavior i.e. lack of following through on seemingly promising words that are spoken, it bothers me to be anywhere near him, let alone try to sleep beside him.

I telephoned Aggie Chretien that day; she is the wonderful masseuse that I had mentioned previously. I left a message wondering if she had any openings, if not, I said that I would book later. My muscles felt sore and I knew this to be something I had neglected to get help with for many months. I hate wasting money and I figured I'd spent enough on metal detoxifying saunas. I hadn't heard from Aggie for a couple of days, so I figured it wasn't meant to be.

That next morning, my hip was so gone that my right foot was not straight. It seemed assembled sideways. I thought this hip displacement had passed. Consequently, I was not feeling any male support, so I wasn't surprised. After I got the kids ready for school and drove them to the bus. Then I drove to Victoria Ave. Since I was nearby, I decided to go for a long over-do walk. It had been a long time since I exercised; after all, part of my job is to increase my bone density. Yes, I forced myself and it turned out to be a joke. About half way through my short walk, I finally let it into my brain that I really was not capable of walking. I was the broken marionette again. All I could do was hope that I could get back to my car without falling. You should have seen how slowly I went over ice and snow patches, but I made it.

CHAPTER 16

Therapeutic Touch Practioner Works On Self

When I got home, I lay upon my healing table and I did a little self-energy work. I must admit that I had sadly lacked the practice this year and then I sat up. I cried loudly and profusely; my arms reaching toward heaven. But I'm not asking Him to take me home. I'm simply telling Him that I think I'm alone. I mean sometimes you wonder; what's the point of coming to a planet with other people? We shouldn't feel alone so much. I guess that's where angels come in; but really, I think people can do better. True, we must be alone to contemplate and realize whom we are, what we need to do and where we are going, but honestly, sometimes life can be so brutal. It doesn't matter what you have, what you look like or who other people think you are. Everyone in life has their struggles. They are just at different levels. Consequently, life can also be so amazingly beautiful and believe me, I have found both in the course of the same day. This day is no different. As I lie on the healing table and continue to work on myself, after my emotional outpouring to heaven, I hear in my head with clairaudience, "Someone that you love is going to call you." No more than one or two seconds later, the telephone rings. Needless to say, I am shocked and curious to see who is on the other end. It's Aggie, my dear masseuse friend. She tells me that she has a cancellation at 2pm. I tell her that I'll take it.

It's nice to get those shimmers of light in the darkness. My mom says that she'll pick up the kids from school because I'll be a little late coming from Tilbury and I am grateful. Aggie worked on my incredible sore spots, I even talked to her about the ones in my heart, not physical. On the way home from Tilbury, I hear with clairaudience that the kids will have some good news about school that day. You would think by now that I would believe in what I heard.

But no, I'm still surprised when my son tells me that he stood up for himself to a bully and he got a friend to do it with him. They chased the bully in the schoolyard until she said she was sorry for being mean, that it was her own fault. And I just now found out from my son, that his reply to this was, "It was all of our faults." It's amazing.

CHAPTER 17

Other People's Thoughts; Know Thyself and Listen

The next day, I become aware of something else. The vitamins that Wendy had ordered for me under the advice of a retired naturopathic doctor, who lectured at a seminar on the weekend at the hair analysis laboratory in Toronto, would be in soon. This doctor figured that the majority of our metal retaining problems lay in the fact that the children and I are severely zinc deficient. My Calcium was too high and not getting into my bones. The London dentist surprised me, months ago and said the same thing. This man said that it was because I was deficient in Vitamin D. Wendy proposed me to him, as her prime concern and bafflement, I'm sure. The thing is, this guy actually believes in M.S., he hasn't clued in that it is related to Mercury and that I was exposed to this poison in large amounts, starting as a young child. The funny thing is after I talked to Wendy on the phone, my legs physically felt worse. I began to wonder if it was my imagination, but I knew it wasn't. Two days later, when she broke it to me about the Dr.'s opinions, I knew she had to be holding the same thoughts about me. If I didn't get better after all these vitamins, it was either arthritis or M.S. I became aware that the negative beliefs others hold toward us, somehow affect our well-being. That is unless we show incredible strength and be incredibly positive even in the face of doubts. I have discovered that sometimes people we think are with us 100%, may turn and cower, live in the tribal thought pattern, abandon us, our knowingness and leave us to be alone. But we can do it on our own; earthly speaking, follow our hearts, walk without doubt, believe in what we've learned and ask those angels to walk with us. This is where I am. I am writing this on Jan. 18th, 2003 feeling better, quite a bit and being incredibly gutsy.

I must conclude with the events of Jan. 16th. I was practising for church. It is the most beautiful psalm. I feel every single word of the psalm to the depths of my heart. Here is the response. "Here, I am Lord, Here I am Lord, I come to do Your will." It was Thursday night. My husband had been so helpful to me that night and so great with the kids. I practised after they went to bed. My husband did wood work in the garage. Actually, he was staining the wood. On the 17th Scott confessed that since the furnace in the garage had been on, he is glad that the house didn't blow up while we were sleeping at night. He said this because the vapors from the stain, he found to be ominously strong. I was shocked and concerned when he told me; especially considering our children's bedrooms are nearly right above the garage. But I held it together. I thanked God and told my husband he needs to listen to that little voice inside his head when he has feelings like this. I'm glad I was praising God that night. Well, I guess I am anytime I do that. On the 16th I sang the psalm over and over. Once again I couldn't stop until I could memorize and recite the entire psalm while immersing myself in it. I had tears in my eyes. I was crying. I made my way upstairs to our bedroom and began calling out to God, "I love You, I love You."

I was crying happy tears, not the kind of tears that I thought I would be crying this week. I got in our room and had to fall prostrate on the carpet, crying and feeling such love for God in my heart that I couldn't contain it. I was bursting with love for God and I felt great. I hadn't felt this intense since Oct 15th, 2002. Though that day was different because then I felt His presence unquestionably. It gave me comfort that He was with me in all that I had been through. Because of that day, I know this and I continue to hold that in my heart. I prayed nine Our Fathers, all with deep reverence. I do love You God. May Your will be done through me. I thank You for this life and for those I love. Be it Your will, may the world and all the people in it be filled with peace. Amen.

What can I say? It is Jan. 21st. I couldn't fall asleep last night and a couple of hours later, my brain brought me to the conclusion that maybe the reason being that I have consumed too much Calcium lately. I had read in a book that too much can cause soft tissue damage, if the Calcium is not making it to the bones. I had thought about my consumption of 'Glutathione' for two months and how I had not been feeling better, only worse. I stopped a couple of weeks ago but since that time I began taking 'Citracal,' which are Calcium tabs. A retired naturopathic doctor had seen my hair analysis and informed Wendy that my Calcium was high and yet he recommended flooding my body with 6 Calcium tabs. Some other good vitamins as well he said are, 'Zinc Citrate.' He said that I, and more so my children, were severely deficient in this. But I know that Aluminum prevents Calcium absorption. I also know that intravenous chelating with E.D.T.A. pulls Calcium from the blood and it is proven to help osteoporosis.

I have been researching again and I am so thankful for the knowledge, but I am sitting here stunned. I am stunned that I have been doing all the right things. I quit eating sugar and foods with additives for over a year now. And, I ate quite healthy before that anyway. I have never been a junk food junkie. Now I learn that elevated Calcium causes depression. Why would I continue taking six tabs per day at anyone's advice? Four days is enough. All I know is that my fingers and now feet are going numb, mind you different than any feeling of numbness that I've ever felt. It is not as severe. I feel like I just found the proof to support my own knowledge. It is the holy grail of Pamela's body. Yes, it's the detective in me again. I know the Zinc supplements will help me and the kids but Calcium, I feel I'm being told to stop. I want another hair analysis immediately. I have to know the status of my Aluminum. Did it change? I also want to lift weights. It is the only way to build bone mass. And I.V. chelating, I am considering. Lead me God, I'm open if this is what is necessary for my healing. Mostly all I can think is that I want to help my children too. I hope the Zinc will help. Actually, I know it will. I can't believe that I read less than two hours ago that Aluminum is less of a neurotoxin than Mercury but it appears to be more persistent. Its physical effects manifest only after being held for a long period of time. I also read that people with cold hands and feet don't absorb Calcium like other people do. The "Raynaud's Disease," I have had since teenage years. I prefer to think of myself more like a temperature chameleon.

My hands and feet are popsicles in the winter to the point of sheer pain and burning hot to the point that I can't sleep in the summer. In the summer I sometimes run cold water over my feet in an attempt to cool them off so that I can get to sleep. I.V. chelating is supposed to help "Raynaud's Disease" too. Do I feel myself being directed? Let's see another hair analysis and my physical body show me if it's healed. I know that the "Raynaud's Disease" is no better. This is a fact. O.K., my story writing has turned into thinking out loud with one's fingers.

Yesterday, Jan. 21st. I lay on my healing bed working on myself, I looked at the clock and it said 2:30pm. I'm certain that I look what I'm sure is ten minutes later and it is 2:52pm, I have never had that happen before.

CHAPTER 18

Incredible Faith Experience

Later at night; I lay in bed relaxing, preparing for sleep. The children are asleep. My husband has gone to help his brother. The animals are downstairs, as usual. Suddenly I hear a noise that I've never heard before. It sounds like someone moved something. It is momentary tapping and clicking; strange, I've never heard that before. Judging by the location in my room and the sound that was made, even though it is dark, I have the feeling that it could be the wooden cross necklace that a few months ago, I had draped in a diamond shape over the top of the brass crucifix. I pull the chain on the nightstand lamp. I look at the crucifix and the wooden cross from 'World Youth Day.' It looks the same. I decide to investigate further. I get out of bed and somehow my left foot gets caught in the sheet. I fall to the ground, flat out again. I am not hurt at all. It was a peaceful fall. I look up and laugh at myself because somehow I have fallen beside the crucifix and wooden necklace on my wall, in a sideways but prostrate position. I am so curious to see what sound the cross makes when I tap it against the wall. I am a little amazed that when I do this, the sound it makes is identical to the same sound that I heard in the silence five minutes prior. In my recent life God and the angels have given me comfort that I might know that I am not alone. I might appear weird, but perhaps Jesus is letting me know too? I remember thinking earlier that afternoon when reading about "Georgette Faniel" that it was Christ she felt closeness to; the Father she felt was stricter. I had been thinking, in my life I couldn't figure that out, my perceptions were opposite to her religious perceptions. But perhaps that is the basis of life's journey, perceptions in the individual soul. Perceptions are unique to each of us. We are all alike, but different. We each come for individual experiences. No one can live life for anyone but we can believe in him or her. We need to allow for that and accept each other where we are.

CHAPTER 19

Irlen Syndrome

Yesterday, Jan. 22nd, 2003, I pick up a 'Tranquil Planet' magazine and the first thing that I read is about children who have difficulty reading and spelling. It's something called 'Irlen Syndrome' and it can be helped by using color overlays. It has to do with altering the brain's perceptions. That night, Daniel happens to pour his heart out to me. He tells me he is the worst in the class. He's not smart, he says. He's never gotten a sticker for spelling dictation this year. I tell him how smart he is and that he fit the profile of a gifted child at age two or three. I know him that well. I finally proved that. My husband finally got some proof when my son started to play the piano. But now, once again, Scott says just to let him be. But he is in pain, it is not I to shove stuff under a carpet and pretend nothing is there. And I let my husband know that. But once again, I'm on my own. I am following my heart while at the same time using my intelligence and my intuition. If I am wrong, I have no problem with that. But, I feel called to do this. I have to try to help Daniel because he is beating himself up. I know where that can lead. I will not stand by idly. Really ironic, it is right beside the ad for the "Enuresis Treatment Centre," the program Daniel had to go through to cure the genetic bed-wetting. In itself when cured, changes the programming in your brain. My husband and his family have trouble with their reading. It is not a judgement; it makes no one better or worse. It just is. But why won't Scott deal with it, if there's a way we can help? Oh wait, I know, it is not free.

I booked an appointment this Tuesday for Daniel to get tested in the Windsor area, so we'll see.

CHAPTER 20

Please Hear Me

Anyhow, I had my own appointment booked for acupuncture at Wendy's on Victoria Ave. A Chinese lady was coming from Toronto to do the work on me. I had put my name in months ago. Today was the day. I think I got her partner instead. She asked me questions about my symptoms. I was happy; I told her that I had no more numbness. She kept telling me about my numbness. "It's gone," I said. She told me my endocrine system needed help. I told her that my gynecologist had thanked me for healing myself. She told me that I could get a different doctor. I was getting angry inside. I thought, "Why did I waste my time and my money?" I know myself better than anyone. I know now this kind of therapy has done all it can for me. I am chelating metal intravenously, I need to be patient or accept my fate. Either way, I know it's God's plan. But the lady did give me a nice Chinese massage. It felt good and I learned my own strength and to not let another speak of things I have wrong with me when I have worked so incredibly hard to be rid of them. No thanks. I have come too far from that little girl who wouldn't speak up and stand her ground, except to the safe haven of her mom. This soft-spoken Chinese woman proceeded to tell me that I was pretty as she worked on me. This is kindness if she was sincere. Of course I told her that I was the little girl who always thought she was ugly. I guess I was trying to say, "It doesn't matter to me what people look like; it's who they are that matters." Understandably, she couldn't read my mind. She told me to, "Cheer up," even though I wasn't sad.

People can't control how they look except in part by the means of what they put into their bodies, but that is a challenge for many as well. No doubt because sugar is addictive, when you start to taste it, you just want more. I think it has to do with coming to grips and allowing our feelings to surface as well. I care about taking care of myself for how it makes me feel. Like I tell my husband, he doesn't have to worry about me looking at anyone. It is a person's soul that I feel drawn to. I had been drawn to his. I hope he doesn't feel the opposite of the unconditional love he gave me. I do tend to keep calling him on the issues of following through on his words and that I perceive he is a workaholic. I guess I am just feeling very strongly about what matters in life, but also I know I need to accept him for who he is. I have to remember my belief of, "What you fear you draw near." I just can't help myself but occasionally to bring up intimacy is really, "In-to-me-see." And I want to see into him but I guess I must be patient first for him to see into himself.

In retrospect at the moment, my lower back doesn't need the incredible pressure on it that my husband so kindly will do for me. I used to need him to push so hard, it caused me a lot of pain but it lessened the pain I was enduring. Seems not to make sense but it's true. So Lily did do a helpful thing for me, besides strengthen my own sense of knowingness.

For some strange reason, I fell again, yes another time. The last time! It was dark. I thought our dog was the cat. The cat does walk right in front of me but at least he gets out of the way. Guess what, it wasn't the cat.

Gosh, it must have been really dark. I don't understand how I did this. Nor did I understand why it happened. It made no sense. Our dog never sleeps smack dab in the middle of the tile floor. When I hit the ground, I felt my brain do the hokey-pokey again, but I didn't hit my head. My elbow hurt but I didn't drop the glass that was in my hand. I somehow managed to hold it up above me while I was falling. Go figure. Anyhow, the next day at church after the, "Alleluia," my mom noticed that I was holding the wall. I had no recollection of this whatsoever. This made me realize that I put something out of place again. That's pathetic when you're getting used to it. I began to realize that my right foot was out sideways again when I walked. Thus, I went to the chiropractor this Monday morning. Ah! I complain about the money but yes, they help people.

It's Monday, my mom told my doctor about my heavy metals and that I was thinking about chelating I.V. This is one of the reasons that I'm so near to tears. If I need it and it will help me; if it's God's will and this is a part of my story, O.K. But really I've been through enough and I think I want a normal life. If God wants me to go through this, then so be it, because I'll offer it up. But at the same time, I've told Him if He wants me to do other work for Him, this is making it really hard. I walk like a drunk. I feel like I could fall any moment. That's fine, but Good Lord I have changed, because of You. I've gone from 'off-the-beaten-path' to not even on the same continent. And I thought most people would consider me unique before.

When Jim McLandress told me on Sunday if I went to Hollywood that he'd be my agent; I thanked him and then I told him that I didn't think I'd make it there because I loved praising God too much. What I mean is that I don't think I'd enjoy singing as much as I do in church. Singing to God brings me joy, that's just how I feel. I had to say that. It just came out because I love God and I know how much He loves us. I want to share that. But where do I go from here?

Here's an idea, I can bloody-well stop waking up at 5:30am, 5am or 4:45am and then not be able to get back to sleep even though I'm still tired. I promise God. I'll meditate routinely every night. This has been going on for a week again now. I want to sleep in until 6am please. When my days have been as such, I'd like a better night, please.

I went to church Monday night, I was going to go with Daniel, and then he decided to stay home. I went by myself and I needed to. It was either that or I had to fit in an awesome cry. Actually, I thought I'd probably do both. It turns out that listening to readings, praying and singing two beautiful songs and receiving the Eucharist helped immensely. I loved the closing song, which talked about God being with us always. I felt at home. I guess that I really needed to go. I was just happy to go to church. I needed peace, prayer and togetherness, especially in this world that I feel so often alone; especially with what has happened to me this year. No wonder I feel alone, like anyone but God could understand me. This must seem ludicrous. Thing is, it's not. I love You, God.

I must have been meant to go to church that night. Otherwise, I have never seen a reason that the children would both part with me so easily.

Scott left to make an ice shanty after I came home from church and this helped me to have some moments alone in order to release some pain. I had still been sad but then as I lay there in bed; I began thinking of the most challenging and beautiful moments of my life. I thought about doing 'Therapeutic Touch' on my Grandpa Vsetula two weeks before he died. This was the last time that I saw him. I was eight and a half months pregnant with Samantha and he was in the hospital. I simply had to go to him and Scott came with me. He was sleeping. I didn't want to wake him so I just began a treatment. Within ten minutes, he was looking up at me with the most beautiful, big blue, happy eyes. He reached for my hands and was smiling. My Grandpa, a man I have adored since I was very little, but also not your touchy-feely type of guy. I can only say that it's a memory painted gently and vibrantly on my heart. It's the last time that I saw him and he died exactly three days after my daughter was born. The memory of doing 'Therapeutic

Touch' on him and the look on his face, made his unexpected death easy for me to take. I was glad he was no longer in pain and I had my little girl with me at the funeral. I suppose like I was the only child at my grandma Elizabeth's, his wife's, funeral.

One more memory that came to mind is my husband's baffling dream. We were married a couple of years and I still remember the night that he suddenly sat up straight in bed, still sleeping. I asked him what he was doing. He didn't answer, but he proceeded to beat on me. I made a run for it. I was screaming. He was beating on me. I turned the bedroom light on. I defended myself; I started to claw at him. He finally woke up. It turns out that he was dreaming. I was a ground hog in which our dog Mocha had fallen in the hole and apparently in the dream; I, the ground hog, was attacking her. Let's just say I was mortified and slept with a glass of water by my bedside for quite a little while. I was afraid to sleep beside my husband. But, he never did do it again. I guess there is more than one good reason to have had our son go through the 'Enuresis Treatment Centre' to cure him of bedwetting and the deep sleep disorder that my husband still has.

That Monday, this memory from two months ago and yet also our wedding day found me lying there in bed laughing uncontrollably. It felt so good. My friend Cindy from nurse's college called me back about I.V. chelating to give me information since she used to work for Dr. Beattie. She told me that when at my cousin Neil's house, which she previously moved beside, she saw his older brother Frank, also my cousin. They apparently were talking about me. It probably had to do with my Christmas newsletter. Frank, who is eight years older than me, said all he remembered about going to my wedding was Scott's brother Chris crying uncontrollably, whining and complaining about me taking Scott away from him. He remembered that no one made him get off the stage. I told Cindy that's all I remembered about my reception too. I remember no one got up to say anything about me at our wedding. When Cindy told me this, I was so happy that someone else had the same experience as I did. My husband had acted like what his brother did was no big deal, it only happened because his brother was drunk. That however, doesn't explain Chris saying to me on the morning of our wedding by phone, "At least he didn't call you fat." I never have been obese. I told Chris in the past that Scott called me a whale when swimming.

So, when Cindy told me this about the whining and complaining, I could just imagine Frank saying this and I had the best laugh that I'd had in a long time. I couldn't stop laughing. It was fun. The memory of Frank's recollections that night found me laughing uncontrollably again. Something I've been doing a lot more since I got my Mercury amalgams out. I love life. I wouldn't have said that with how physically bad I was feeling two hours ago. Isn't life great?

I am writing today because I had the best sleep that I have had for at least one year, and that's even with the kids waking me twice through the night. I had a good sleep. I didn't even hear Scott come in at 1:15am. But, I took the longest meditation that I've had in a substantial amount of time. I know I haven't been giving it the time necessary to make it a good experience. What I did get from the meditation is this. I've been told that when my healing is completed, life will be a fruitful experience. This is brave to say in my current state because right now I don't actually know God's plan for me. I have endured so much. The meditation taught me that the healing is because of Love of God, wisdom of the body, truths of the mind and strength of spirit.

CHAPTER 21

'Irlen Syndrome' Results

My mom, Samantha and I took Daniel to get him tested for 'Irlen Syndrome' yesterday. While I was there, it was as if time stood still. It was a vortex of learning for the three of us, including Jo-Anne, who was the assessor. I felt like a fly on the wall, in charge of occasional documentation. The revelations that took place with Daniel brought tears to my eyes at one point. I could see the difference in my son's comfort and behavior when the colors best for him were discovered. Daniel's self-knowledge played a major role in this. It's amazing when you follow your heart and are open to the will of God. I learned about 'Irlen's Syndrome' last Thursday. The following Tuesday; it's proven present in my son.

Listen to your children, people. We are all in this together. I talked to my son at bedtime. In the morning he told me that he told himself he was smart two times. He didn't want to do this at night but I had him repeat this and explained my feelings about myself as a little girl. He did not think he looked any good either. I never told him that this is what still touches a nerve in me. Part of the reason is that when his daddy saw the 'Teacher's Toy' commercial that the three of us were in, for the first time; that it hurt me so badly, almost like a knife when my husband looked at me and the first thing that came out of this mouth was, "That's a bad shot of you." I knew it wasn't a bad shot, but I immediately thought I must look ugly. My husband said this to me when I was so excited to show him the children and me together. I hadn't even planned on being in the commercial. I only thought it would be the children. Later, my husband told me that he was jealous. I thought, "He's my husband, isn't he supposed to be proud of me?" It took me a while to get over this. Sometimes I think I'm still working on it, to be honest. I realize it challenged my own sense of self and my confidence. At least my husband said a feeling he had. But am I a hypocrite because I told my son last night that he holds the key, when he starts to love and appreciate himself, others would also? I love myself more than I ever have and the criticism can still get to me. I don't think that I am being hypocritical, I think it hits extra hard when it comes from the person you most expect support from. But we are all human and on some level, I can put myself in my husband's place and understand. But at the same time, I can't stand the idea of speaking before you think. It can be so hurtful. I have been challenged this year; but I'm positive and it's getting better.

CHAPTER 22

The Birth of Daniel

After a 57 hour labor and still unable to sleep after his birth, I was grateful that Scott was there to pick Daniel up when he needed feeding and changing. I remember the time that Scott slept in the hospital bed with me after I had Daniel. I was grateful. Ironic really, when I was pregnant with Daniel I thought he would be a girl, until the last two weeks that is, when I heard Elton John's "Daniel" song on the radio, then I felt/knew different. My main gift in parenting this child, I felt, was to be of help to what I previously thought was a little girl. I thought I'd be able to help this child with her life, so she wouldn't have to endure the pains I did without anyone to truly understand me. But he turned out to be a boy. Even when I had him, the nurse said, "It's a girl, it's a boy." That was strange. And it is within my little boy that I view some common threads between him and myself. I didn't know boys could be so highly-sensitive. I guess it is how they are raised and I am glad to raise a boy with feelings. If he gets married some day, I bet his wife will appreciate it. I already appreciate it. My children are compassionate when I get hurt. Also, in Daniel I see qualities and strength displayed by him that was nowhere near me at that age. He's teaching me to stand up for him and thereby myself at age thirty-two.

Jan. 29th; I took two Calcium pills this morning, I felt I should. It has only confirmed that this stuff is not helping me. I feel worse for it. It's taking all the patience that I can muster to wait for the hair analysis results. Either way, with research and my own personal hell, I'm leaning the direction of I.V. chelating. Over the last month it is going down the stairs that is giving me great difficulty. If I didn't hold the railings later this morning, I know I would have fallen, and as it stands, I'm lucky that I accomplish that when I feel this poorly. This only occurs when I go down the stairs. Does that make sense? No. It barely makes sense to me and I'm living it. My right back hurts so much. But get this; I'm only numb when I take Zinc or Calcium pills, in my hands yet. No, this hasn't happened before, only when I began these vitamins. My system is still faulty. It has to be. Otherwise your average human could handle vitamins. Are the metals still present? I am tempted to give it a resounding yes. Either way, I offer up this suffering. I still have trouble understanding my husband not understanding me. He told me last night I should come ice-fishing. That a little fresh air would do me good. I suppose this is what it is like to live alone in one's body. No matter what you say, no one can understand? Maybe that is why people like disease names. They have to have this in order to compartmentalize people. Sorry, not me. My faith won't let me. My brain and heart agree.

CHAPTER 23

Prayer for All and What Mercury Does to Hair

I pray for peace in these questionable times in the world, for everyone. May love devour fear and may everyone's heart be open. Amen.

This same question comes to mind on occasion, "God, why am I writing this and why can't I stop?"

Another thing, how does a girl whose hair has never ever been curly in the wintertime get that way? It is pulling the amalgams out. The week that I got the last one removed; is the first time my hair went curly in the winter. My grandma had curly hair, I inherited it but it was hidden under my poisoning. My eyes; they were as blue as my daughter's until the third grade. Then, I tell people, they changed color. This coincidentally was the time that I began to get the strongest of my toxic fillings. The irises of the eyes display toxins in the system, i.e. browns and yellows. My eyes were very blue as a child, but at the age of eight, they seemed a funny green. There are brown rings around my pupils. The funny thing is, I am not the only one who noticed my eyes changing color for the better this fall. My son, about a month ago, told me that they looked blue. My husband said that they looked clearer; they lightened up. This has become obvious to me, especially since I have spent my entire lifetime looking at them. The changes are measurable, just like in my hair. In these trying times, there are days this is all that I hold onto, my hair and my eyes. I also remember how much lighter my face felt when I got my first three amalgams out. I could never have imagined the possibility that such a small measure as taking the metal out of three teeth would affect the physical feeling in my face. You don't have to believe me, I am the only one who knows its truth. Granted, I am sensitive.

I have learned one thing. Suffering is not an obvious thing. We need to be good to each other. We need each other in this world.

Well, just as I heard last week, the hair analysis came in today. Wendy told me that the levels were normal. When she called me and told me the numbers, I told her it still sounded high to me and that I did not feel normal. As it turns out, when I picked up my results, the Mercury was even a little higher than it was with the original test in the summer.

This made sense to me considering the truckload of amalgams I got out. There is no doubt also, considering my symptoms after getting them out. Also I have read, Mercury is inconclusive on a hair analysis. The analysis, I believe, only measures organic sources of Mercury, not the inorganic sources. The silver had come down incredibly. I guess it is an easy metal to dispose of, that and I had been taking homeopathy, Argentums, for that. The Lead came down a little and I took homeopathy for that too. The Aluminum came down from 13.89 to 8.63. It is still by far my highest metal. I came across an article last week that states 'though Aluminum is not highly toxic until the levels become high and have been there for a long time, it is one of the most difficult metals to get rid of.' Most of my symptoms include lack of balance. I think a drunk would look more sober, paired with lack of muscle control i.e. it's almost as if they have a mind of their own.

Along with my dizziness; it matches with the toxicity symptoms of these two metals. I also find it fascinating that my Calcium is not as high, but still quite high, especially for a girl with holes in her bones. I believe the Aluminum coming down has allowed for more of the Calcium to be absorbed. I checked out the ratios between primary and secondary, most recent, hair analysis. I compared Aluminum readings to the Calcium ratios. Aluminum was 1.71; Calcium was 1.2. Pretty much in sync, especially considering Aluminum must leave first before Calcium can be absorbed. Remember, premature osteoporosis is linked to Aluminum toxicity. Thus, completely of my own devices, I have decided to go the route of I.V. chelating, unquestionably. I will call tomorrow. This of course does not mean this hasn't ripped me apart. I do wish it were all over and I had no more to endure, but when getting through every day is an incredible test of strength, at the same time I'm glad the analysis came up as it did. Yes, the saunas and homeopathy brought the metals down, but for the work I did and the consistency with which I have aspired and lived; these results are not good enough. Do I wish I did it I.V. in the first place? Yes, I think so if I knew how it would go in the end. Yes, I thought I could get away with saving more money, being in town and taking less time away from my family. As it turns out, the answer is no. But life is a learning experience and I know things happen for a reason. I would not have learned what I did if this wasn't the case. Besides, I spent enough time running to London to get my teeth properly treated. The present moment offers me the time to go near London again and at the same time not put myself through incredible rigorous treatments all at once. I was not pleased with my friend Wendy trying to talk me into the fact that things are better. She was sugar coating to put it nicely. Doesn't anyone have compassion enough to get with my soul and see what I've had to endure? Right now all I need is someone to say, "It's awful what you've been through," and give me a hug. But so be it. I definitely am going to meditate every day. I will not miss a beat; it is too important and feels too good.

I thank God that my cantoring practice was delayed until this afternoon when I got my hair analysis results. I sang to God and I felt it all. This coming Sunday's psalm, "The Lord the valiant in war;" I can relate to it. However, mine is not your typical battle. The following Sunday, the last I'll cantor before going on holiday for a week-"Praise the Lord who heals the broken-hearted." I was almost in tears standing up there singing today. For that matter, I was almost in tears when I pulled into the church lot. Thank God for all those beautiful children to sing with. I've been at the point lately that when I put the dishes in the dishwasher, I sit on the ground in the kitchen. My back has been aching so badly, I'm dizzy; this is equalled only by emotional turmoil today. But I offer it up. I held both my children in that kitchen today, grateful and needing their hugs. I can also relate my walking and stair climbing experiences to the little engine that could. I am just not over the hill yet, but believe me; I'm nearer to the top than when I started a year ago.

Jan. 30th, I am happy; I slept until 5:55am. I started my homeopathy again this morning. I'm totally going it on my feeling alone. These metals are still present in too large amounts, in my opinion. Since my back and right hip was so painful, I went for a massage. The woman I met said that I had scar tissue over my right hip and the only way to lessen it is to massage deeply with a lot of pressure. This explains how I've asked Scott to massage and push my body so much that it hurts severely, I explained to him that this helps me feel better. Marcy tells me that scar tissue can be disposed of, if worked at. This scar tissue a.k.a. fascia holds a lot of toxins; so I'll take an Epsom salts bath again and drink water with lemon juice. She likened scar tissue to a scab on a cut that pulls the skin but the scar pulls the muscle in this instance. There is always something to learn. What she said finally explained the severe pain in my hip and lower back. I booked an assessment appointment with Dr. Beattie. This puts me on the road to intravenous chelating therapy with E.D.T.A. I see him next Thursday. The aforementioned are the last two avenues, physically, that I'll embark on to cleanse my system, I feel it. This is where I draw the line.

I find most helpful, these words that came to me on Nov. 1st "All Saints Day," 2001. I was told that it was coming from St. Andrew. "Be at peace and you shall receive peace wherever you go."

At this point I'll close, no more writing for a while. I'll leave with what I began my day with, "As morning breaks, I look to You. I look to You oh Lord to be my strength this day."

CHAPTER 24

Prayer for Morning and Prayer of the Chalice

It's a favorite prayer of mine that I've been praying every morning for at least half a year now, probably more. The bracketed parts are my own additions to the author's work.

"Most holy and adorable trinity, one God in three persons, I praise You and give You thanks for all the favors You have bestowed upon me. Your goodness has preserved me until now. I offer You my whole being and in particular all my thoughts, words and deeds (and songs,) together with all the trials (and joys) I may undergo this day. Give them Your blessing. May Your love animate them and may they serve Your greater glory. I make this morning offering in union with the divine intentions of Jesus Christ who offers himself daily in the holy Sacrifice of the mass, and in union with Mary, his Virgin Mother and our Mother, who was always the faithful handmaid of the Lord. Amen."

O.K., another favorite:

THE PRAYER OF THE CHALICE

Father, to Thee I raise my whole being
—a vessel emptied of self. Accept, Lord,
This my emptiness, and so fill me with
Thyself-Thy Light, Thy Love, Thy Life
—That these Thy precious Gifts may
Radiate through me and over-flow
The chalice of my heart into
The hearts of all with whom I
Come in contact this day.
Revealing unto them
The beauty of
Thy Joy
And
Wholeness
And
The
Serenity
Of Thy Peace
Which nothing can destroy.

CHAPTER 25

Hard Times & Good Times

Scott and I had our first huge fight yesterday. Yes, Scott didn't close his eyes and avoid it. And it was still horrible. I couldn't believe what he was saying. It was about the 'Irlen's Syndrome' again. He said, "Let kids be kids," otherwise known as, don't do anything about it. I was totally and completely losing any shred of hope between us. I reiterated time and again that he open his heart.

At one point, I yelled out what he had said to me since he didn't seem to remember what he had said. Then he looked at me and told me that I should be a lawyer. It was almost a compliment. When I'd lost all hope, he hugged me, he picked me up and said that he was sorry and started to kiss me. I thought he wanted something from me but he said, "I just want to talk." Holy Cow! Then we lay in bed and he told me that he wanted to make me happy, he wanted to be a better husband. I was afraid to believe, but he said that he would make the effort. I told him how bad it had gotten. Wow! After this, I thought, "Oh my Gosh! My story, I gave to Father Jim. I knew he had to have prayed for us." I just knew it. I have never, ever been able to get through to Scott before, no matter how nicely I asked. It was like a miracle. So, this morning he and the kids went ice fishing. The phone rang for the second time at about 10:45am. I made it to the phone. I am not fast on the stairs. Before I picked up the receiver, I hear with clairaudience in my head, "It's Father Jim." It was! He said the biggest compliment he could give me is, "Your story is not at all phoney." I thought, "Yes, that's me." But then later, I thought, "Wow, with what I wrote and the strangeness and depth I touched on, that is a huge compliment." He's coming for dinner on Sunday the 9th.

Just now I put the color overlays over top of Scott's newspaper. He said, "It does make it easier to read." I couldn't believe that he was serious. He was. "Yeah!"

So much has happened. Sunday I sang a psalm, the 24th, only the words that I sang had war and armies in it. These words aren't even in the 24th psalm in my Bible. These two words, war and armies, only reminded me of George Bush and I don't even watch T.V. to know this. Saturday night when I discovered this, I wished I wasn't doing it. The 24th psalm in my Bible is truly beautiful! The two words I was to vocalize; were not beautiful in my opinion. Of course, I sang it that morning. I didn't mean to be quiet or not pronouncing well, but somehow I did just that. Later when I told my mom my feelings about the words, she said, "I was surprised by you. The words are so easy to hear usually." I had to laugh at myself, what I did without realizing.

Saturday night had me questioning what business I had going on a trip in my physical condition. I lose my balance and fall. Thursday night, I could barely walk and went to bed at 8pm. This is so freaky, I don't understand. But wait, it gets freakier. Sunday, Scott and I went out for dinner. Five minutes after I got in the restaurant, I started to get stomach pain. I hadn't even eaten anything or drank. Then, the longer we were there, it grew excruciatingly worse.

The pain was unquestionably in my stomach. I offered up my pain to God and I did energy work. It didn't change much. I told Scott that I had to leave, but I had to sit there and watch him eat dessert while I endured. When I got into the truck, it still hurt, but I didn't have to lie down on the back seat as I anticipated. When I got home, I went straight up to bed. It was slowly getting better. Within fifteen minutes, it was completely gone. I went downstairs. It never came back. I haven't been losing my hair this week. For two weeks, whenever I took a bath, I would see a bunch of hair that I would leave in the tub. I could not figure this out; it had never done this before. Well, it has stopped for about a week now.

I talked to Mary, she called me and she told that me her hair was falling out in clumps, big clumps. I was curious about how long it had been like that for her. She said, "Oh, about two weeks." Her doctor is testing her for Lupus; apparently she has a rash on her face too. I have got to come clean and say, "I do not understand my life, but I love it. I do not understand what is happening to me."

I am taking Iron in a liquid supplement. The last hair analysis that I had shows that my Iron is incredibly low. It has never been like that in my life. But my Mom read in my Mercury book, it's at her house; that Mercury pulls out Iron. I guess that would explain it because I have had no recent haemorrhaging in the last six months. I am happy that I am getting a menstrual cycle. This is three in a row. Today, I got one, 28 days after my last. In my life I haven't ever been that regular that I could predict the day that they would come. I am not having any pain with it either. This is miraculous.

Another miracle is my son reading with his color overlay on his French book. He told me that the one he picked was too hard. Then he read it and got through it like I've never seen before. I've never recently had a day that I would call typical and that I didn't learn something or get pulled into a different experience. This, I had never anticipated. I pray that prayer every morning!

Last night at church was amazing, "Amazing Grace!" I put down my book and I sang all five verses from the heart and listened to readings about faith and a sermon about life's challenges. Amen.

CHAPTER 26

Domination

So much has happened. My husband came home from work on Tuesday, right after 4:30pm, I might happily add. I was getting the children to clear the toys from their closet and bring them down the basement. I had also been working on a totally homemade apple pie for Sunday. I asked Scott to carry Daniel's giant chest of Lego down the basement, kindly as usual. But then he had to ask me a tonne of questions; why and why Daniel couldn't push it down himself. I didn't feel like building a case. Then he started to ask me more questions about things he could throw out, like the new book holder that I purchased for $4.00 because it helped Daniel to read more easily. Only Scott wasn't holding it when he asked me the question. I informed him of that and I got called a lawyer for the second time in our marriage and within the course of one week. Is this funny? I wish, I became unbelievably stressed; I desire peace, harmony and working together. Probably the reason that my husband decided to take his anger out on the cat after I asked him ten times; this is no exaggeration if he'd put Daniel's chest in the basement. I would if I physically could. Back to the cat, he was only sitting on the stool by the phone. He hadn't even attempted to jump on the counter from there. But Scott couldn't find the squirt gun, so he dumped a glass of water on Sage. The next morning, I smelled and discovered that it made kitty pee when Scott had soaked him. I spent the evening cleaning supper and pie mess, music practice and telling my hubby that he doesn't have to threaten the kids to make them listen, and not with the spanking again. It began to hit me that night, why would my husband grab my hands while I was peeling apples and start saying, "No, no, Pam put down the knife." He said it joking, but creepy like. The week before, he grabbed my hands in the same way. When I held a lighter in my hands ready to light a candle, he said, "No, no, put down the lighter, don't do it." As I lay in bed early Wednesday morning, I began to ponder this. What was he trying to do? This was not funny, kind of sick actually. Wednesday morning, I had not been feeling well. My physical body is not working easily to say the least. I asked Scott to drive Daniel to the bus. He came home, without argument, and stood waiting as I finished Daniel's late preparations. He didn't say a word to help me or to encourage Daniel to respect me. I let Scott know how I felt with the lighter and knife episodes. I was angry and not being my best with my son. I let my husband know again that I needed him to parent with me. Scott called at 9am to apologize. He said that he was sorry for being a 'butt.' I had been very upset and I was crying. I was thankful for the apology but asked him if he called to say that he was sorry because he thought I wanted to hear that or if he really realized he'd done something that wasn't right. It sounds picky, but when you don't know if your husband is even aware of what he does or says, you have to ask. I am so exhausted from being hurt. But I was so happy that he had called, it gave me hope. My day would have been tremendously worse otherwise, and it got bad anyhow.

I followed my mom's wishes and went for a Vitamin B12 shot. I prayed before, asked for some saintly help and I was in and out of the doctor's office in 5 minutes. This was right before it got busy and I didn't even have to see the doctor. My first ever B12 shot went well. I felt perhaps a little better, but it wasn't the cure. I am mostly vegetarian so I understand, I may be deficient. I went to the health food store for a few groceries and ran into the chiropractor's wife. I was introduced. She asked me about my amalgam removal and if I felt like a new person. I told her no, not really. She suggested other things to me. I told her that I have researched and been involved in solving things myself. When she questioned emotions, I informed her that I have dealt with that. I have been a busy and aware girl, you know. I was glad to see she was picking up on that. Such that she respected where my life had led me; the wisdom that I've built upon and she said; "You look like you need a hug." I was so happy, just what I've been hoping for and from a total stranger. "Let me know how the chelating was," she said and I wished her well. Another high point of the day, my daughter came and gently took my hands so that we could dance to 'Mama Mia' together. I really had no business going to choir, I could hardly walk at this point and was very dizzy but I love to sing with the children. I heard other's hardships and it almost brought me to tears for the realization of myself being in such a boat and yet at the same time for the pain others were enduring. What made me most sad was that I wasn't well enough to offer Therapeutic Touch as a regular service for these people. I wanted to help them.

We met Scott for supper, fast-food, after choir. Daniel wanted to get his spelling words done. Scott started to ask him a word and, like the night before, I offered to Scott how it was pronounced since he did not change it; I reminded him since this is how Daniel's teacher was going to pronounce it. Scott for the first time asked me, "Well, how do you know it's the right way?" I was surprised, he knows that I took French until grade thirteen and it is just something that I've always been good at. I told him that I trust him when he's good at something like his work. This took another small chunk out of me. Doesn't he trust me and know me by now?

CHAPTER 27

Funeral Singing

After singing at Ursula's funeral; I realized that I didn't know her, but I liked her. This was only by reading her obituary and hearing about her. She endured 103 years on this planet, so I felt compelled to honor that and sing at her funeral. I loved the songs that were to be sung. Though Marilyn told me that I didn't need to be there, I had to go. And after asking, I found out that Ursula did pick the songs. They are my absolute favorites. We sang; "Amazing Grace, Prayer of St. Francis and How Great Thou Art." I sang the last two to my babies from day one and the first one most recently and often.

CHAPTER 28

Chelation Centre

After the funeral, my mom met me at church and we went to the 'Southwestern Ontario Chelation Centre.' I had an E.K.G.; some other preliminaries and then I met with Dr. Beattie. We talked a good while, lots of metal and medical jargon. He even checked out my teeth and said I have some metal on one. I had never looked because I didn't expect any. I will have to question the London dentist. Anyway, Dr. Beattie is great. And he feels with my symptoms that it is Mercury causing the problem. He took six or so vials of blood and agreed with me that it was extra-cellular and that nothing would probably show up. Until that is, he is chelating me intravenously with E.D.T.A. and does the urine test to see what was flushed out. He tested my muscle strength too.

I awoke at 4:50am this morning and felt that I should be chelating Monday before the trip so it's good to go. I am listening to the angels who turned off the kitchen light last week, the split second after the thought of chelating the day before the trip entered my mind.

CHAPTER 29

Barbados Experience

We just got back from Barbados last night. What an experience. This was spiritual beyond my wildest dream, yet soul ripping. My physical challenges made last year's trip seem like child's play. If I had had a laptop computer, I feel I would have been writing for a good deal of my vacation. I am having trouble typing this morning because my fingers are numb inside, but this is par for the course lately. Upon getting on the flight, I had a feeling that the person I would be sitting beside would cause spirituality to come to the forefront. The level we attained; was unfathomable. I listened to her life story. She searched in her Bible and passed on four beautiful psalms to me. I wrote down their numbers. She even told me that she came across something she had never noticed in the Bible before she met me. I told her some of my experiences and she prayed with me, aloud on the airplane. I don't think she quite understood where I was and I had to tell her that I had already given my life over to Jesus but I thanked her that what she had brought me was a renewed hope for my marriage. She said that she had had a nervous breakdown with what had happened in her life and that her marriage had been rebuilt, even though it still has challenges sometimes. Her husband is a West Indies diplomat. I have so much to write but am having such a difficult time getting my hands to move where I want. Celia Bullen had asked God to sit her beside someone who needed to hear her speak. I told her my feelings about something happening. This happening on the airplane made our five-hour ride seem like moments. I knew God was telling me the trip was meant to be. I am grateful. I did not ask what religion she was, it did not matter; she loved God.

I made an appointment for a massage as I was physically having difficulty the next day. The woman who came, Rita, told me that she expected to have an old lady as a client that day, just the feelings she got as she knew not why she was coming to my hotel room other than for a massage. It was like meeting an old, dear friend. Our views on the world, peace, and people were so similar. She was from Iran and spoke that nothing has ever been solved by war. She had lost family members when Iraq invaded Iran and wanted no one in the world to have to go through what she went through. I agreed with her and talked further in depth. She told me that she worked on two 'White House clientele' that did not want war. They knew that if they didn't do what they were told, someone else would. At least these men cared. She said one of their wives was crying as the man spoke. She said though they had nothing bad to say about the president; neither did they say anything good about him. I could not believe that she trusted me to share this. At the end of my massage, she told me that my legs needed deep muscle massage, as the muscles were extremely tight. I was glad that she noticed. She looked surprised that I gave her a hug before she left the room. Our special connection had meant that much to me.

We ended up at 'St. John's Anglican Church' again, this time at Samantha's request. This will be our third year, first in 1991, then 2001 and now 2002. Scott headed toward the backyard cemetery of 'St. John's' with Samantha; the whole reason being that she wanted to go, this was with Daniel too. I went looking for the gift shop; pretty ironic considering that I purchased absolutely nothing on our vacation. On my way I saw a man in a makeshift wheelchair. He appeared to not be able to speak and he kindly pointed me toward a door. In my head I wondered why he was in the chair and for how long. I with clairaudience receive; "He has been struck with polio as a child." I am surprised to have this come to me as I am not used to getting information about others. I prayed for him. When we are ready to leave, I get brave and search for proof. I ask Ian, the man who made Scott's necklace, about the man in the wheelchair. I need to find out if what I heard could possibly be correct. I knew I had to take the opportunity and ask. That's life; there are choices to make. We can seize the moment or we can regret listening to the inner self. I will not opt for the latter anymore; it is too painful. Ian tells me that the man's name is Charlie and that he left. I ask him why he's in the chair. He tells me he heard that he has been in the chair since he was very young and that polio struck the island. I am awestruck. I never expected it to really be true. Another confirmation that I should stop doubting what I receive?

It is Wednesday morning; I am sitting in order to further recount our vacation. It hits me. I am poisoned with Mercury. It is bad today, very bad, I can feel it. Mercury causes a low White Blood Count; I read this and had put the book down. It feels like someone walking over my grave again. That is what my blood test showed two weeks ago, my count was 4.4 on a scale of 4-

11. I cannot do anymore. My hands won't work. I am finding it difficult to type with any accuracy or speed. I quit.

It's Wednesday afternoon, it's 1pm, Holy Cow! I've realized; I know what is wrong with me, Mercury poisoning! It is something only God and I know because at this time, I have diagnosed this myself. I have had moments of fear today but now I stand strong and unafraid. The funny thing is, as you read on; my doctor gets behind me and supports me in my knowledge, he offers me further chelating. He offers me his treasured book on "Amalgam illness" to read. I saw Dr. Beattie's book, which was written by a Harvard doctor. God gives me confirmation; support that my diagnosis is correct. Every symptom of mine is in that book; symptoms I have had since teenage years. If you want to find out, keep reading!

I'll flash back one week, Wednesday in Barbados. We got together again with Leo, under the stars. The entire day consisted of thick cloud cover but I told Daniel that we needed to thank God in advance for the clear sky, so that we could join Leo with his high powered telescope as we so enjoyed his Wednesday show last year. I told Daniel that it was going to take a miracle to get that sky cleared up. It happened, the show was possible. We could see the stars. Leo is a brilliant astronomy buff. I knew him intrinsically in a way that I did not know him last year. He showed us Saturn, you could see the rings perfectly; something that after this year will not happen for a long time.

I told him that it was stunning. I told him that last time we were in Barbados; he inspired us to teach our children more about the stars. He said that he wished there were no lights in the city; then the beauty of the stars would be radiant and obvious. I knew from that moment on that Leo was a highly sensitive person. When the presentation was finished, Leo handed us a copy of a newspaper article he was in and he invited our family to come to his house sometime for a private show. The man simply loved what he did. I read his article before bed that night. My husband had suggested that I take a look; he said that he knew I'd like it. I was surprised. Leo was into E.S.P. and liked to do healing work. With this trip I became keenly aware of God's presence offering confirmation.

It's Thursday in Barbados. We spend time on the beach. I'm glad that I brought my rosary, when you can't walk without losing your balance, it leaves you time to lie on a lounge chair, catch some rays and inconspicuously pray the rosary. Sometime during this beach afternoon, I become aware of some knowledge that surprises me. Yes, I heard clairaudient words. They are not your own thoughts, not your words; they come from outside of yourself. That doesn't however mean that you aren't going to doubt their authenticity.

I hear that I am going to give my story to Father Joseph. It surprises the heck out of me. I can't believe it. I think, "Yeah right, expose my inner most personal self, not knowing how he would take what I know. Many others would deem this unbelievable or weird." I question it and think that maybe it is my own thought; even though truly I know that it's not. So I say to myself; not out loud of course, "O.K. you want me to do this, offer me proof." Minutes later I hear with clairaudience, "You want proof, you will hear the name Joseph a few times tonight." I laugh to myself and think, "Oh sure." Dear Father Joseph, if you do end up reading this; please know that I am not ill in my mind, I thank God for that. I have complete compassion for those who in their lives must endure these trials. After having a semester on the Psychiatric ward in nursing, I swore I would never use the word crazy because it is condescending and hurtful to those who live with mental illness. I must say that I have faltered and still occasionally use this word in the place of silly. I hope you can decipher that clairaudience is to the ears as visions are to the eyes. My son and daughter can attest to seeing 'colors' that most adults and children don't see. My son has even shocked me once and described an angel sitting on his bookshelf. It was sincere. I don't see, but I believe. Boy, I sure am bearing my soul. You must understand, I needed some proof since you are the priest that I sing God's praises in front of every week, so I did not wish to harm this relationship. What happened that Thursday night? We went to David's restaurant in St. Lawrence's Gap. I take my daughter to the teeny tiny bathroom and there's a poster map of 'St. Lawrence's Gap' on the wall. I examine it and see at the bottom right corner, a little restaurant named 'Josef's.' Moments after I spot this I hear with clairaudience, "Your daughter is going to point this out to you." So she gets up from the toilet in a couple of minutes, looks at the map and the first thing she does is point to a 1cm square block with the name 'Josef's' on it and asks me what this is?

I tell her and think, "There's the start but it is still not enough to convince me." I guess that I need a lot of proof for this one. After a lovely dinner, the chicken is different than at home. The difficulty began mostly because my husband remarked that the chicken was boneless. This freaked out my son, even though I cook this kind at home. He was mortified that chicken ever had bones. I talked to him with much calming and convincing; we all ate, then left. We are walking back to the hotel, not the cab this time. I use the term walking loosely, but not as loosely as I will at the moment I am writing this. We get a little ways and my husband points out and remarks, "There is 'Josef's' restaurant." I had told him, an hour earlier that Samantha pointed it out on the bathroom map. I am surprised that Scott spoke so vibrantly about this, but I am still not convinced of any proof since I did tell him about it. I read to the children about St. Caedmon as a bedtime story since I brought my book of saints with me on the trip to read and I found his story so easy to relate to for children and adults. I think this is the night that I also read to Daniel from his confession book, which I purchased from Sister Mary Diane. We love the story of St. Francis. Minutes pass, stories are over, now the lights are off. We lay in bed. Daniel pipes up from his bed and the first thing he says is, "What about St. Joseph?" I am startled. I inquire as to what makes him ask? He says, "How come he was the only member of Jesus' family that didn't ascend into heaven?" After talking, I lie there and think, "I'm convinced. You got your point across three times and I know it." I reflect and realize it's about God's will being done, not about me. Though I can't see how my not-so-little story could do much other than alter someone's view of me.

So I ask my husband if he would mind if I gave my story to Father Joseph? He said he wouldn't. I have only given it to six people to read, and at no time was it ever as forthright and open as this account. It has evolved and it has become incredibly open to the details of my experience. I sincerely doubt that even in its safely held-back versions, that even one of these people could believe or even remotely understand me, let alone not think me odd. With this you will know why I was adamant about proof. For goodness sakes, I am the woman who's greatest love is for singing at the church, praising God because He has my undying love and my soul felt a deep resonance the first time that I ever heard about Parish Nursing after reading the London Diocese paper.

It's Friday in Barbados, the first day we rent a car. I had plans to go for a drive but something else happened. A woman commented on hearing our children playing violin and piano the day before and was appreciative and very complimentary. She told me that her and her husband's friends were meeting them at the hotel. She said that the man played piano by ear. She invited me to bring my son to meet him and play with him. My change of plans threw my husband but I explained it was an incredible opportunity for Daniel to meet an adult who played by ear. Daniel was up for it too, so we hung out by the pool until the noon meeting. It was an incredible time. Daniel played and Charlie was impressed and so kind to my son. He kept asking him to play more. Daniel played; 'Amazing Grace' and Charlie broke out in song.

CHAPTER 30
Barbados Experience Finally

The other couple, the man's wife and I joined in too. I asked Samantha if she would ask her dad to get the violin. He did and then she played with her brother. Then Charlie played. One of his songs was, 'How Great Thou Art.' I was stunned and so happy. We were all singing. Even my husband quietly joined in. The two men, Charlie from Winnipeg and the other man from Cape Breton whose father made violins and whose mother was an orchestra violinist, had incredible voices. My husband has an amazing voice that I would love to sing with too, but he prefers not to do it together very often. What an incredible experience. We broke into song in the piano lobby of this peaceful, floral and tree laden, environmentally conscious hotel. Our second year at the 'Casuarina,' the hotel with the mission statement proclaiming protection of the earth by the conscious awareness of our human actions such as composting, no chemical cleaners used and an ozone pool with minimal use of chlorine. It was a blessing to have it brought to my attention last year.

The rest of Valentine's Day was tremendous as well. Dinner at the Crane Beach where my husband and I had been on our honeymoon was great. This was a definite highlight of my trip. It was kind of funny. I couldn't walk straight. I drank two glasses of wine but it didn't change what was already there. One woman gave me a dirty look as I went to the bathroom because I lost my balance and hit the pillar. I said out loud, "I walk this way when I am sober too."

We went to St. Thomas' church on Sunday. Half way through, I found out it was an Anglican church. The sermon was an hour, the service three hours. The pastor's sermon completely resonated with me, he said we are like athletes and in God's service; the most difficult time comes with physical weakness. I had to agree. He also talked about the need to look at oneself, saying that the biggest fool is the fool who isn't aware of his own foolery. The pastor asked the visitors; which was our family only, to introduce themselves and say where they were from. It was great, he asked the children to come to the front too. Daniel with a lot of reassurance; went to the front of the church with the other children to receive a blessing and two cookies. We saw Samantha kneeling before Canon George. Apparently this church used to have only fifteen people. Now with the current pastor, it had about two hundred. He was amazing to listen to. Now, I knew why I had felt the inner call to attend this particular church so far from our hotel. I needed to hear his words, they offered me comfort and my husband was completely into it too. It got his attention. It was a neat experience. We were the only Caucasians in the whole church and we didn't care and neither did anyone else. I needed to be there to have comfort; as I told my husband, because Saturday when we went to the animal reserve, I could no longer physically walk after I persisted through the weaving and dipping stone pathways. I had never gotten to that point, but neither would I give up. I became aware that other women would probably have asked their husbands to carry them; not I, I would not give in. I would not succumb or faulter. I did have to sit down while my family went on to look at plants.

I regained my strength, at least somewhat, from the level to which I had sunk which was the bottom. I had not been able to walk, not even a few more steps.

Now I could make it to the car after a rest. That night, it hit me. I thought about what I had endured physically. It took all my strength and energy to walk, keep my balance and get through this vacation. As I lay in bed that night, I honestly would not have cared if a stranger came and stabbed me in the heart and killed me. It was that hard!!! I don't recollect if I even hoped that someone would put me out of this. Thank God for sleep and faith.

I was physically in deep trouble Monday. I could hardly walk and lack of balance was brutal. I lived this. I asked Rita if she could do massage or reflexology. She came to my room a few hours later and proceeded to tell me to exercise regularly to build my strength. "Oh no! It's another one. Okay, I am getting used to this." I explained again that it was the Mercury. This trip caused me to walk more than I ever had in a year. Things were only getting worse, but I was glad to have confirmation that my condition was in no way due to physical muscle deterioration. She told me that three women on the island had M.S. and had their amalgams out. I couldn't believe what she was saying, that these women would know it was related to their condition. She told me that it was actually an herbalist who told them to do this. Then Rita told me that since she had seen me the last time, she had done research herself and had made an appointment with her dentist to talk to him about getting her four Mercury amalgams out. She confided in me that she often had a metallic taste in her mouth. She told me to be careful and watch what I used and ate so that I didn't put any more Mercury into my overloaded system. I told her that I was doing this already and that I had done ample research. I left her Dr. Beattie's business card, telling her that if any of these women with M.S. would ever like to get the medication mailed to them that helps the body dispose of Mercury, I thought it might be possible. I left her my name and address as well. I told Rita that if she gets her amalgams out, that she should eat certain things like free-range eggs which help the body chelating heavy metals. When she left, I stood at the kitchen sink doing dishes. I was in shock over what Rita told me she was going to do. I looked up and told God out loud, while smiling and sort of laughing, "You're starting to freak me out." I was coming to the belief that He was using me, as I so often wished, to help others. I said to Him, "Your will be done through me."

As I walked to the beach, I saw a woman by the pool in a wheelchair. I wondered if I was ever to talk to her. It bothered me to see her suffering like it bothered me to see an older lady a few days earlier, ambulating stiffly and laboriously. I will never forget that evening, as I held my husband's arm while walking down the street. He turned to me and said, "It is really a struggle for you to walk, isn't it?" I felt my eyes moisten. I told him, "Finally someone understands what my life has been like in the last year, and it's you!" That comment from him, changed everything; it gave me peace and hope. I so appreciated that he had been pulling my chair out before dinner for the first times in our marriage. This vacation changed our marriage.

My husband had to be there with the kids because he did understand what I was not capable of at these moments.

Even Fern's comment, about me being a crazy one, after I confessed my toxicity to her, didn't bother me in the long run. I simply had to say that I loved her for who she was and the gifts that she had brought to the children in wanting to hear them play their instruments.

On the beach later that Monday, while Scott had taken the children further down the beach, a youthful man drove his wife onto the beach in a wheel chair, beside me.

I wondered if I would somehow be given the opportunity to start a conversation with her to understand her story and offer compassion. I watched, my heart full of compassion and sadness, as he picked up his wife and brought her to the water. He stood her and she leaned against him. Her body reminded me of viewing a saint's incorruptible body, but she was alive, though one could scarcely tell. She couldn't make use of her arms and barely her hands. He brought her back to the chair and she began to video him in the water, though to me it looked as if she was going to drop the camera in the sand. I asked her if I could help in any way? It was difficult to understand what she was saying, her speech being affected as well. Her name was Sue. I offered to take video of her and her husband and they were happy, as it was a rarity for them. Thing is, I was kind of afraid to hold their camera, afraid I would lose my balance. After I found this brave person inside me, asking her how long she'd been in the chair. She said, "Five years." Later I asked if I might know what put her in the chair? She told me Multiple Sclerosis. Though I know I already knew the answer. She told me about how she woke up one morning and thought she'd had a stroke. She was paralysed on one side. I told her how hard if must have been to go through what she'd gone through. I told her a bit about my last year, so she would understand some similarity and then I knew in my heart that I had to tell her about heavy metals. I wanted to plant a seed of what I had learned in a chance it might help her. I thought myself pretty brave or nuts considering the current state I was in. But, I had to do it! I also did not want her to feel alone or different, just because of her appearance. She suggested to me to see a neurologist. I told her about Dr. Beattie and the chelating that I was about to undergo.

CHAPTER 31
Home, Chelation Resumed

Thursday, I am home and it is chelating day number two. I am extremely ill. I can hardly walk. I get the kids to the bus stop but for the first time, I won't get out of the car. I am so tired also. I am blaming my husband for awakening me again at 5:30am but today, which is Friday; I had gotten up at 5am on my own and fell back asleep. When I got to Dr. Beattie's, my mom had to give me her arm so that I could walk safely up a tiny snow bank. I was open about the poor shape I was in. That's how bad it was. I talked to the most amazing older gentlemen after an hour had passed. I finally felt like sitting up in my chair. I asked the nurse for my Mercury blood test. While I was waiting, I was informed with clairaudience that even though I thought it would be zero i.e. non-existent in my blood work; it would in fact be apparent in my blood. I was afraid to hope that what I heard would be true, but I shouldn't have been. It showed up as a count of 5. Proof for me that I could show others it truly flowed in my system. It really doesn't mean much I realize, this is nothing as far as in blood, I know it is in my organs; intracellular, but some extra cellular proof was just that. Mercury is a stinker for showing its presence; it is like a silent invisible phantom, killing you by slowly sucking the life out of your body. I realized that I have been brought to this physical incapacitated level so that others might see what Mercury is truly capable of. I make no softened statements. It is hell. But I offer it to heaven. I am sitting here today incredibly dizzy, barely able to balance and all I can think about is that I don't want others to go through this, diagnosed disparagingly and incorrectly.

Dr. Beattie, I thank God, offered me his self-proclaimed Mercury Illness bible. The knowledge within this book written by a Harvard doctor is incredible. This life I have been living so alone and so darn certain of my

Mercury poisoning which I have self-proclaimed in the last two days with not a seed of doubt in my mind, has just been handed to me with further proof that I can provide to others in book form. I am going to order it myself; but for now I devour the book. I even managed to put some dishes in the dishwasher this morning. My husband took my son to school, I had to explain to him that the dizziness wasn't off and on, it just was. And my mom told me to rest, she worried about me all night and all I can do is to sit here and write. But hey, my fingers are typing this morning. I am on a pill, after telling Dr. Beattie how I couldn't do up the buttons on my daughter's sweater yesterday. After that, he saw that I could barely walk or balance. He gave me the green light to take D.M.P.S. This is an oral drug for chelating Mercury from the brain. Upon questioning him, I found out that I.V. will only chelate the blood, but this pill will pull Mercury out of the brain. Kind of ironic, I did not know this when I was confessing to Dr. Beattie that I could not get my fingers to do what I wanted and I told him that I felt this to be a function of the brain. You get what you need. It is so nice to be heard. He told me that I would probably feel worse before better, but my mom and I had the same thought; how could I get any worse? Believe me; I know this is courageous to say, "You shouldn't ask for, what you are not prepared to receive."

But, truly I am not afraid. I had reached the bottom of a barrel that I was certain I had already found. On the way home from Dr. Beattie's, I was so grateful for my mom's presence. I physically felt that I could do nothing but lay. I sat in the car while my mom got the kids in the school.

As I sit here now, I feel energized inside. Yesterday, I felt frustrated. I have nothing but self-assurance and confidence in what I know. Personally, I am going on complete trust in God. It's hard to explain, other than to say that I am listening and I have faith. It was hard to convey this to Marilyn on Wednesday afternoon at choir practice, before my Thursday chelating appointment with Dr. Beattie that I had told her about. She suggested that I get to a doctor in town. I realize that I am probably freaking her out. Heck, I openly told her the Wednesday before I even saw the Harvard book that I have Mercury poisoning. For goodness sakes, I don't know everything, but I have a passion to learn all that I can. I want to help people and I better include myself, so that I can do this. I do research. Do people think when you are an at-home mother; you sit around and do nothing? I would not claim to know what I know if I had not the grounds to do so. Doctor's are not God. They are human. My dad, I would say, also gives them super human prowess because they are medical doctors. I respect the vast training that they have undergone and in an emergency, there is nowhere else that I would rather be. There is a time for them. I wanted to be a physician, before I met my husband. Does not someone who is a nurse, who got the proficiency award hands down, out of eighty people; deserve a little respect for knowing the boundaries of the medical profession? I believe in prevention and not being satisfied with a disease label. We need to find out the causes of these diseases and fix the ones that are fixable. I'll go out on my limb again and say that there are many. And I will be forthright and say that drugs don't cure but allay the symptoms. I believe that we need to search deeper and deal with how we take care of ourselves. Do we have the gusto to do our best for ourselves? If not, fine. I accept where others are and what they have come to learn. Please accept where I am and that I've chosen to do something for myself on the premise of self-knowledge and faith. We can't possibly truly understand someone else's life unless we hear their feelings. We can listen and give them credit for where they are at in life. I can't say that I am ever stagnant, I allow self-introspection, but I am never stagnant. I was thinking about Jesus a few nights back and how much pain He must have been in to say, "Eloi, Eloi, lama sabachthani," meaning my God, my God, why have You forsaken me? It was incredible beyond words what He endured. I imagined what His passion must have felt like. Barely imagining it was painful. But what he went through! I wanted to get mere glimpse, so that I could convey it when I sing the psalm, "My God, My God, why have you forsaken me?" I had to examine this, because I could not feel easy singing these words that at this time I would find challenging to say to God because of my faith in Him. But thinking about what Jesus endured, it leaves no doubt in my mind why He uttered these words. I thought about His passion and undergoing my circumstances yesterday, this to Jesus would have been a speck of dust compared to what he endured.

I felt I got a glimpse in the slightest manner. I thought about His closest friends around Him and His mother, not one could do anything to alleviate His humiliation, belittlement and excruciating pain. He chose to do God's will, offer His life as a sacrifice and He still does offer it every day. I have heard of people asking for the blood of Christ to be poured over others to protect them when they were suffering. I told my husband, I didn't think this right. I will not ask Him to suffer anymore for reasons that would seem petty. We as humans need to make our own efforts, follow His example, pray and be thankful to Him. There are saints who have offered to live His passion to help other souls. Do we want to call on their sacrifice if not absolutely necessary? Let's help each other in this world. My mom is so incredible at doing this. She is quite a woman, selfless and giving, to animals as well. Though I am not completely understood, I have not been alone even though I have often felt it. I thank God for light in the darkness. God has incredible timing.

During our I.V. chelating, Murray, Clark and I talked about how medicine can become about keeping pharmaceutical companies in business, not getting people better. These men dealt with angina that is cured and not by some magic pill covered by O.H.I.P. but by chelating that they have to pay out of their own pockets. Apparently the current U.S. Vice-President at the time I write this; has undergone this treatment and has improved his health. They aren't conveying it openly on the news but finally their medical system is doing a serious investigation.

Dr. Beattie told me that the woman who was diagnosed with Lupus was there at the same time as me on Thursday, Feb. 21st. Let it be known that Lupus was a label put on this woman who instead is cured from what was truly Mercury poisoning. Chelating cured her. We will meet when the time is right.

CHAPTER 32

Kindness

On Friday, I pondered my singularity and aloneness in my medical preventative focus. My dad offered me emotional support. My dad! He did this by simply mentioning his doctor's appointment this week. He saw a physician who was filling in for his physician. She is my doctor too. He said this man was Chinese and preached to my dad about the lack of necessity for drugs. He told my dad that if everyone would eat healthier by watching what they put into their body and if they exercised; that there would not be a need for pharmaceuticals. Wow, an M.D. and he is speaking this aloud to his patients. It is great. I really am not alone. Perhaps just not in the majority. But then again, I found that in my new friend Murray as well. This is the man that I met at the 'Southwestern Ontario Chelation Centre.' Murray is a retired teacher, as is his wife. We agreed that life is not about following the crowd.

It is Saturday. I am singing the 41st psalm tomorrow. I found out the number by the book Jennifer gave to me. Seconds ago, I read it in the Bible. It is incredible. God has amazing timing, amazing comfort and amazing friendship. I love You, God. The intimacy only You and I know. Thank You. Praise unto You always. Praise to Jesus Christ. I give love and honor to Mother Mary. I give gratitude and reverence to the Saints. Holy Spirit, I have yet to discern between You and angelic communication. I guess that I have only to ask, call on You more.

I am glad that God loves me. My husband makes me wonder; this must be what happens when you don't even examine your own actions. I am very ill, can hardly walk and have eye and headaches. I am not capable of doing much around our house, let alone with the children. But my husband leaves for work on Saturday at 6am and says; "See you soon," all sweet and honest like. I hear from him at exactly 2:45pm. Maybe he is truly intuitive. Yes, that's it. He knows even though I'm on oral chelating drugs to remove Mercury from my brain for what will only be three days that I am not in danger of adverse reactions. Even though yesterday, he got upset at me because I was laughing at myself. He said, "How can you think it's funny that you can't walk?" I told him that I have to laugh at myself and I'm lucky that I can because I know what is doing this to me and that lets me live in hope. That and I trust in whatever God has planned for me. But it's Saturday, obviously he's not a worrier, which is good. Like I told him, I am glad tomorrow's readings prepared me for forgiveness. But I think it is sad when I have to question his love for me. How many times have I told him to just be honest with me about when he'll come home? I'm not into false, decorative baloney. For some strange reason I still trust what comes out of his mouth. I have asked him nicely. That reminds me of my son, whom I tried to help with his French homework today. I talked nicely to him. He didn't listen; he kept telling me that I didn't know anything. He was in Grade 2 and I was in Kindergarten. I had to tell this boy that I was smart. He told me that I wasn't. I tell him that I took French until Grade 13 and got my first and only trophy for getting the highest marks in Grade 8.

He continued to run away from the table, threatened and started to do his homework in ink. My mom was there; she saw first hand and offered me support after I gave him a gentle slap on the cheek. I am not normally physically punitive, I don't believe in it. I don't want to bury a child's emotions. I figure that this is what happened to my husband. I only want to live through kindness and honesty. It is how I prefer to be treated. I prefer to not be emotionally abused either. I am realizing now that I have to do this myself also. Scott won't talk firmly and strongly to Daniel when I ask him. He doesn't seem to know what to do since I've pleaded with him and he finally listened to stop threatening to spank the children if they won't do something he asks. Isn't life an interesting school? I always said that I like to learn. However, I am not sure just how many courses that I signed up for at the same time? Talk about balance! I could use that (Ha Ha!). I'm feeling that when I lose the Mercury at least physically I'll be there. But emotionally, I laugh. From where I am at today, I think about Celia and she says when there's trouble in your marriage and your husband seems to fight you on everything, tell the devil; the actual devil, she wasn't talking about one's husband, to get out of your house. With how I feel today, I am thinking that I had better ask the angels to intercede every time; before I speak to or am with my husband. It can't be Canada but why on earth was my husband kind, considerate and well-mannered on vacation. I look at myself; I am not acting any different towards him. I thanked him for taking the children to their music practice yesterday when I physically was not well enough. I guess that I am finished pouring my heart out, I think I shall liken this computer to a heck of a large glass. I am tired; the exhaustion comes and goes. To me this is new. I am sitting down and resting in my current state. It leaves me no choice. My sweet mom did laundry, though I begged her not to do it. I know my writing now is taking my energy. But it is a passion. The story that goes, God knows where. Don't you God? I am glad because I don't know its purpose.

CHAPTER 33

Another Mercury Poisoning Symptom

Today is Saturday, Feb. 22nd and I had better close because my eyes are ceasing to focus together as happened to me yesterday. My eyes were obscuring on two different places at the same time without trying. Physically, I am severely lacking balance and coordination, these are more poisoning symptoms; some things are much better than in 2001. For instance, I can go up stairs without dread and mustering every bit of strength I've got. I just can't go down without holding on for dear life. I can get in our vehicle with running boards more easily than last spring. I remember at this time, my husband remarking that I was getting in like his eighty year old grandmother, and he's right, I was. One thing I am certain about, my husband cannot say that eating well and purely made me sick. In Barbados I did not have access to what I do here; I felt the difference. No rice milk, only cow's milk, no organic vegetables, no brown rice there. I feel that my eating habits have sustained me and given me incredible energy to get through the past year. It is only now that I am sitting down and resting. And let's face it; walking and stair climbing only made me grow weaker because I pushed myself so hard. Dr. Beattie reaffirmed that this is what happens. Dr. Cutler's book states, "Exercise mobilizes Mercury and needs to be done in MODERATION." This explains why I got worse as the days went on in Barbados. I was walking and walking, pushing myself to a degree that I haven't in about a year. It explains why going for a walk on Victoria Ave. last summer often left my head spinning for 20 minutes. Two days into my Barbados trip, I developed pain in my left eyeball and a headache that wouldn't leave. I rarely ever get a headache. My eyeball still hurts to touch it or to look downward. The pain makes me jump. This symptom was present in Dr. Cutler's book that was lent to me three days ago. Even athlete's foot, on my left one, so seemingly typical, is a recent symptom for me. I kept wondering why it wouldn't clear up. His book is two-hundred pages, I can't possibly sum it up, but I will order it and I will lend it. This madness needs to stop. Do people need to hit the state that I am in to become aware? Myself, I prefer not to learn the hard way. Dr. Cutler's book about chronic Mercury poisoning is controversial; controversial because apparently if a dentist admits to their patient that Mercury is a neurotoxin, he/she is in danger of losing their license. What a bureaucracy! The only thing that comes to mind is 'Adolf Hitler' and fear tactics. I am sorry; it just popped in. Yes, most people have these fillings. My teenage "Raynaud's Disease;" was my hands and feet feeling like popsicles. I had gone through 'Irritable Bowel Syndrome,' which Dr. Cutler lists in his symptoms of toxicity. I had always had irregular menstrual cycles before Samantha was born. Present symptoms like incredible dizziness, last year's vertigo, my pathetic lack of balance; I sit waving my hands in space to try to stop myself from falling if I go to far out of body centre i.e. if I'm even a little too far forward, back left or right, down I go. I know my root canal that touched the depths of my gum tissue and then proceeded to turn my gum grey in two years was most probably the cause of the apparent sudden illness.

All the other so-called liveable symptoms I had; were apparent since my teenage years, if I dig deeper and examine other Mercury toxic characteristics. I could pretty easily presume that I had them since childhood. I demand dentists to stop using it on children. The dentist in London won't do it. My dentist in town said it's too difficult to put plastic composite in children. Why does a Paediatric dentist in London use amalgams? He will use composite but only if you ask and let your feelings be known. Wait, I know why; Mercury is less hassle for them. If you let your child eat frequent popcorn or hard candy, chances are the plastic filling might sometime need fixing. You will find no one to dispute the fact that Mercury is poisonous. But they think not in your teeth right? They say it is forged; it can no longer escape even though you chew with them. HA! What of the vapor that is emitted when placing the fillings? Denial is not a river in Egypt. I love society. I will not dispute living in the present, it is the only way to go. What if what you are doing stupidly jeopardizes your future or your children's future; all based on convenience? Life is not about living unconsciously; if it is easy do it. We all hold different opinions. People only see what they want to see. Chances are that someone could be a good person, wise and yet people will look for a perceived flaw because it doesn't fit with THEIR belief system. They would have to change, grow or let someone else hold a view that challenges their own. We will never be identical. Be tolerant world! God did not mean for us to be identical. There is not one perfect path that all must follow or they lose. But I am hazarding a guess that we are on this planet to learn from each other. Jesus set the example; that all need to work for God's plan. You need not be crucified as He did. Let us honor and help one another. My favorite thing is people who already have amalgams or whose children have these;. Understandably why would one want to think these might hurt their children? Goodness, my son still has one when my dentist scared me into it before I knew better. The London dentist even used to place them for the first five years of his career. Please don't choose them anymore. Look at the Europeans? Are they paranoid? Do they do things without proof, HA! You see what you want to see until you realize that you are hiding from yourself. My mom tells me that I can do something about this because I am living it. I am open to the will of God.

CHAPTER 34

Urine Mercury Test

Sunday was the first time that I used a walking stick because I had to. Singing to and for God was once again the highlight of my day. Sunday night, I was as unstable as the ball in a pinball machine. Monday was worse, the worst. I was so glad that my mom was picking me up at home to drive me to the 'Chelation Centre' and of course Daniel to the bus-stop beforehand. During the whole drive I felt sick. I was dizzy beyond comprehension, my left eyeball hurt so badly. I was nauseated to boot. How I felt inside was truly indescribable by words. The fatigue that encapsulated me on the way to Komoka was what usually hit me on the way home. I could not wait to get chelating. I knew that the D.M.P.S. pills had pulled the Mercury from my brain and put it into my system.

I needed an extra boost beyond regular kidney function to get it out of my body. It took three tries for them to get the I.V. into my hand. I could care less, this pain is nothing compared to what the Mercury is doing to me. At the chelation centre, I could feel my face and lips gently twitching. This is quite a journey when you can feel it but no one else can notice. I talked to Dr. Beattie. He checked my eyes and refused me more oral brain chelating until he got my urine test. He said, "If it shows in the urine; going by the specificity of your symptoms, we will definitely know that you are a very Mercury toxic girl." I believe, I conveyed to him that I already knew this without a doubt. I could hardly stand in his office, my balance severely impaired and my memory not functioning. I had a brain fog. Perhaps this is the reason that I did not remember to press Dr. Beattie for another urine test. I knew that after my three day Mercury brain digging drug; if it were to show in my urine; now would be the time. But everything happens for a reason. I felt God's call to bring it to my family physician; that she could become aware of the effects and presence of this toxin in people. I felt so incredibly ill, my head spinning and aching, and no strength in my limbs and I was completely nauseated. I did not know how I would even pull off dragging myself into the doctor's office. I prayed to God and I asked 'Padre Pio' to help me communicate with the staff in order to get me to see the doctor promptly, if of course it was God's will. This was the turn around. The most abandoned and worst I had ever felt, did an about face. Even though I could barely walk and stay balanced for the whole day, I declined my mom's help getting into the doctor's office. She got out of the car anyway. I told her that there was a ramp and that I had the walking stick. I told her that I'd be okay.; even though I wasn't sold on what I was saying. When I got in the door, I asked the receptionist if there was a urine test for Mercury. I told her that I'd appreciate knowing. I told her that I didn't come to the doctor's office very often. She said, "I don't know about the Mercury, I'll ask Paula." Paula works for the doctor and gave me the B-12 shot a couple of weeks ago, she is not a nurse but I have no doubt that God worked through her. I heard her get on the phone and call the laboratory to see if they could do a urine Mercury test. I heard her talk and laugh a little. Then the receptionist came back and said, "Yes, they do a test."

Here is a urine bottle but remember you have to wash your hands. I asked her if it had to be the mid-stream urine? She said she didn't know. I asked her if I needed a doctor's order because I had already asked if the doctor was back from vacation yet and she said; "No." She told me that she'd give me a Doctor's requisition for the urine sample. I said, 'Thank you" and went to fill the bottle. I was going completely on inner direction and living in the moment, not even thinking if my bladder was full. Somehow, I even ended up getting the mid-stream urine, though I wasn't trying to, I just couldn't catch the stream at the beginning. This I found to be peculiar. When I got back to the front desk, I asked if she would like me to drop it off at the laboratory since it was on my way home. She said, "Yes, that would be great." I was in and out of the office in 10 minutes. When I got back to the car, my mom was shocked. I told her that God has amazing timing; that it must be meant to be. I was smiling, intoxicated with joy and appreciation. I looked up and said, "Thank you, God."

My mom drove me up to the door of the laboratory, with the children still in the back seat of course, and I got out. A kind woman held the door open for me. Even though I thought someone was ahead of me, that wasn't the case. I was asked for the bottle and my health card. I asked if they did these Mercury tests very often. Apparently, it had been a couple of years since the last one. I asked her if they did a urine 'Porphyrine' test at the laboratory. I had just this day read about this as a very specific Mercury test but the person doing the laboratory work can't expose the sample to light, shake it or agitate it and that it must be refrigerated. If not, what would be positive could show as a false negative.

The other woman working behind the counter said she didn't think they did this test at their laboratory but she got on the phone to find out more. The other woman, who I had handed my basic urinalysis to, asked me why I was getting it done. I told her that I had chronic Mercury poisoning. She said, "How would you get that?" I told her about the numerous Mercury amalgams that I got when I was a very young child. Then I told her that the root canal I had done two years ago; had corroded and turned my gum grey. I told her that this was the one that gravely tipped the scale out of my favor. But what I have come to know is that many so-called diseases, I had gone through; are listed on the front cover of Dr. Cutler's, "Amalgam Illness" book. I graciously thanked the woman who had found out about the urine 'Porphyrine' test. Apparently, they do it at the laboratory. I told her that I would probably go back to the doctor some time and ask to have it ordered. I have a reason for doing all this. It is not for me. I have nothing to prove to myself. I have no doubt in my mind what has caused my life to deteriorate to where it is a massive challenge to function. This proof, I believe, is what is required for the knowledge of others. When I am better and not living hell; they will never forget there was something wrong with me. I am here to help others, since it is God's will. Wherever You lead me God, I shall follow. Thank You for shedding light in the darkness. I love You so much, life seemed so lonely and insurmountable before. I love You so much, but You know that and You know I tell You how much I love You, even in the darkness.

CHAPTER 35
Holy Gratitude

I'm glad that Scott offered to take Daniel to piano on Monday night. I was exhausted. Thank you, Scott. I spent an hour lying in bed with my daughter after our bath. I read some psalms in the Bible to her; the ones that Celia showed me in her Bible on the airplane en route to Barbados. After hearing a little of my story, she thought they would be particularly helpful to me. They are Psalm 34 and Psalm 91. I now know where the song, "On Eagle's Wings" comes from and she suggested Psalm 45 too. She also told me about Ephesians 6 i.e. the armor of God. I read this one to my family in Barbados. I was glad that there was a Bible in the hotel room, my son had to search for it but he found it. Last night with Samantha, I turned right to the 22nd Psalm. I read it and was happy to find it but I was profoundly sad as I read it. It was perfect timing as I recognized it as the Psalm that I would be singing on Monday simply because Marilyn had told me weeks before that I would be singing, "My God, My God, Why have You Forsaken Me." As I read it, my daughter asked me if she could say, "Too bad, so sad." I told her that if there were ever a good time to say it, it would be now. I told her that she could say it all she wanted. It almost brought tears to my eyes; even more today as it was really hard for me to hold it together when I practised with Marilyn. I told her that it was Psalm 22 as she looked for it in the CBW. She asked me if I knew whom it was about; even after I had sung it with her once. I told her that, "Yes, I know it is about Jesus." I must be honest and say that I was a little shocked that she asked me this. Who else would it be about?

I am tired and sad right now. But I have to write. I talked to Dr. Cutler today, the man who wrote the book on "Amalgam Illness." With that book he gave me confirmation when I had come to the conclusion that I'd have to walk this alone at least on earth. He lives in Wisconsin. He picked up the phone and I asked him if I could order the book. I thanked him and said, "God bless you for writing the book." I asked him how we could make dentists stop using Mercury. I asked him if he thought it was a bureaucracy. He said, "Yes, this is a good word to sum it up." I offered that if he ever needs support to put an end to this, that I would be on board. I asked him if he was ill before; he said, "Yes." He told me that the doctors didn't think it was funny when they asked him his symptoms and he replied that pretty soon they would be psychiatric after dealing with all the things the doctors said to him. I would love to meet him some day and writing this, one second afterwards the phone rang. Be careful what you write. When again I sat down, I really did just want to catch up on my writing but it was my cousin Janelle on the phone. Her marriage has broken up in the last year and she needed to talk. We talk longer than 15 minutes.

It's Wednesday. The saga continues. To condense it, I was very ill this morning. My eyes felt swollen. No, I wasn't crying, yet. I had the best sleep in a long time but somehow I was exhausted and very nauseated. I made it to drop Daniel off at school and to get Samantha to her violin lesson.

In the middle of the lesson, her teacher asked me more about the symptoms of Mercury poisoning. She said that Jordan, a teenager who plays violin and one that I took my first and only water color painting class with; had a mother who can barely make it up stairs and falls all the time. The doctors have no idea what it is. Kerri told me this. I told Kerri that the lady could call me sometime if she wishes. God knows I'd be happy to help. Afterwards, I went to my doctor's office to get a phone number that Dr. Beattie can call for my urinalysis results in case his results aren't in. I was stuck waiting for 45min. this time. But a woman I had gone to high school with, asked me about the cane. I told her my story and my viewpoints about giving Mercury fillings to children and she said that she thought I was smart and that is something she definitely would not give to her two young children now that she knew. She encouraged me to keep it up. Then my aunt, Janay's mother, came in. I talked to her and was glad to give her a hug. I knew that she'd be very sad as Janay's birthday and mine was only two days away.

God kept me there so long for a reason. In the afternoon, I began to write on the computer and just got a sentence out that I wished all of this stuff would stop happening so that I could get a break. Earlier at the doctor's office, when I spoke to my aunt, we talked and talked. She ended the conversation saying that she always felt so uplifted when she talked to me. She helped me too, reminding me of the importance of couples having time alone together. Scott called to see how I was doing too. I felt optimistic, other than feeling physically ill. I can only say that I cannot surmise the rest of my Wednesday in a positive light. I came to the point, only half an hour ago that truly the rest of the world does not care what anyone else is going through because what's happening isn't happening to them. I feel more like a clown in some sideshow. I don't feel believed. I was so incredibly dizzy at choir practice, my balance brutal and my head throbbing softly with pain. I was glad to sing, "On Eagle's Wings" and I was happy to tell Eric that the words from the song came from the Bible. He seemed surprised and repeated what I had said. When I got home from choir practice, I told my husband that it hurt to move my eyes. He told me to close them. This hurt my feelings; all I asked is for a shred of compassion from the man I love. But then I hurt his feelings because I didn't like his comment and he said that he wouldn't talk anymore. I apologized to him. I realize that the pain of this afternoon had come unleashed on him when he said those words that I so desperately hoped would be caring. Later, my husband suggested that I go to a neurologist. I know, I know, I must not appear to have a shred of knowingness or intelligence especially to those closest to me. I underlined my symptoms in a book and I told him to stare at my lips when I opened my mouth to see if he could see that they had a tremor. He could finally see; I showed my son too. My husband finally hugged me an hour later. I think the fact that I was crying for half an hour helped too. It gets totally disheartening when you go through stuff that no one can notice. I have begun to conclude that most people are blind or either too wrapped up in their own world to notice.

Though I did get a hug from Cheryl at church, after the funeral this week when she listened to my story after inquiring about my cane. But basically I feel like I scare people. I don't know what they think about me? Right now, I am the one who is scared but not because I can't handle what I'm going through. No, more because I'm tired of going through it alone. I spent the last hour talking to Jesus because at least I know He's there. Someone else was there too, my children called me from Scott's mother's house after their ice cream. Daniel was first. He was worried about me and told me that he loved me; then Samantha came on with the same sentiments. They were so compassionate. Now that was true love, the sustenance of life. I needed that. I appreciated that.

I will not be bashful; going through the last year or so has been a living hell interspersed with glimpses of heaven. It's only that I keep trying to put my bravest and best foot forward that perhaps no one can tell. Funny, I thought the pain would be written all over my face. My God, how much can a soul endure? My husband asked me tonight what I wanted for my birthday. I told him that I wanted a friend. That is all I want. I am not being selfish about it. I give what I get. I care about people. I love You God. I love You Jesus; I am so sorry that You had to go through what You did. Let the world remember You and what You came to teach us.

CHAPTER 36

Compassion

It's Thursday morning, February 27th, 2003 at 5am, my last day of being age 32. I awoke and felt dizzy in my head as I lay in bed; I knew I wouldn't be able to sleep. I was nauseated. This is the first day that I've awoken and started to cry. I am talking to God; asking Him what is going on with my pain? I get back that I won't be given anything I can't handle. In my head I hear that the world needs this right now for the state that it is in. It might sound crazy, but I have told God that I offer Him my life. I am still crying but I tell Jesus that I offer this up. I am told to get up after half an hour and then I get a rosary to pray. I hear my husband get up downstairs. I go down and realize that I need to talk to him, to try and put some of the misunderstandings at rest. I tell him how I feel because he asks. I tell him that I only want him to understand why I react as I do. I told him it was very nice of him to buy me flowers late last night with the children. I explain that I was not extremely thankful because when the children called me and were genuinely concerned about me, I could hear him talking and having a good time in the background. I didn't even know he would take them visiting after getting them an ice cream. He had already spent half an hour talking to his friend on the phone before he left. I explained to my husband that I did not mean to be ungrateful. It was just that 'worldly things' didn't matter to me; truly I only desired friendship. And the thing is, being physically alone doesn't bother me, but emotionally is another story. Last night I tried to explain to him and he kept telling me what he did was never good enough for me, what he said was never good to say. I asked him if he ever noticed what came out of his mouth. He only keeps telling me that he loves me after all this. I get to the bed; he is in the bathroom and I start to sing the song, "More Than Words To Make Me Feel That Your Love For Me Is Real.

What Would You Say, If They Took Those Words Away? Then You Couldn't Make Things New, Just By Saying I Love You." I tell him that I am not perfect. I am sorry that he feels hurt. He asks and I tell him that many times I've already told him what I need. For goodness sakes, I was so thankful five days ago when he finally read this whole story; what I'd written so far. Now he just calls himself a 'smuck.' This morning, I am very calm as I speak to him. I tell him that I am not complaining about the fact that I am poisoned. It just is and I offer it up to God. I tell him that I will get better. I think about the prayer of St. Francis and I tell Scott that I know it is not as important for me to be understood as that I should understand others. Somehow, we end up talking further and Scott tells me that no one can be my friend or talk to me because I won't listen to their suggestions. He is angry when I told him that my eyes hurt. He feels that I made it difficult by being very hurt when he told me to close my eyes. I told him that I only needed some compassion and understanding like, "Oh, your eyes hurt?"

He seems to be blaming me; I tell him that I accept and look at the things that I do wrong. I am not perfect. Did he ever hear what came out of his mouth? We talk more; on his way out the door he tells me that I am high and mighty.

The comment just about kills me. I say, "Pardon?" not believing what I heard. "You think you are high and mighty," he repeats and continues saying that, "You won't listen to people telling you their suggestions as to how to get better." I explain to him that it is my body; that I am living in it. I said if there were a doctor who had done as much research as I had; and truly understood what I had and how I felt; I would gladly hand it over to him/her. Still I have the grand honor of not being allowed to know anything. I asked Scott if I question him as to whether it is truly his gallbladder that hurts when he is in pain. Then he walks out the door and says, "See you later honey, I love you." This seems to be going from bad to worse. I told him last night that I have so much love in my heart to give. I asked him if he did. Considering we both claim the same feeling, why is it we appear to be on different teams? Gosh, I shouldn't expect too much. It's not like I am used to it. Though I thank my dad for all he has done for me financially, worked so hard and given so much to his children. But depth of feeling or compassion from a male figure has not come to be something I expect. Maybe going through the most challenging time of my life and reflecting on the marriage vows: "In sickness and in health," has caused in depth thought. The importance of true depth and intimacy has been thrown in my face. "Silly Pamela, she always said how much her husband and her dad were alike."

I asked Scott this morning if I were like this in Barbados. He didn't say anything. I continued saying that I could feel how much he cared about me there, we were together and nothing else mattered. Now he seems to be running away again. But I am committed; I will be honorable and let God guide me. Everything happens for a reason, correct?

CHAPTER 37

Ignorance

This is the same day and what a day it is! On the way to 'Komoka' for chelating, my mom tells me about talking to my brother and his wife the night before. He thinks that I need to go to a doctor; he didn't believe that the man that I am seeing is one. His wife tells my mom that I have always been sick. Her kids are healthy and she will continue to put Mercury amalgams in their teeth. The thing that my sister-in-law refuses to look at is that I seemed apparently healthy as a kid too; chronic Mercury poisoning accumulates over a lifetime, every time you eat. As for root canals, I am happy that their children don't have one. They are not putting Mercury fillings in adults the way that they did when I was a teenager, if you go to the right dentist. At least now, once in a while, you are offered a choice, but I believe most dentists will advocate Mercury as the preference. My sister-in-law would also probably not like to hear that her son's permanent teeth became brown, mottled and gooey because of 'fluorosis;' which is fluoride toxicity. This can happen to the baby in gestation or quite simply by letting a child use too large amounts of fluoride toothpaste.

I was hurt by their remarks; it especially hurt because they are apparently concerned about me but never bother to call. Also, they think since I use Therapeutic Touch and am a Recognized Practitioner that I am someone who has lost my intellect and have no medical knowledge. I get zero credit for being a nurse, and as my brother said, "You are not a doctor." My mom told him two days ago that in high school, I wanted to be a doctor and that I would have made it and been a darn good one. Apparently this made my brother stop in his tracks. I have never felt so pained that I would actually say out loud to myself with sadness, "I lost my family." I didn't feel emotionally like I had a brother. But of course, I'll forgive.

CHAPTER 38
Urine Mercury Results

This is the sickest; actually poisoned that I have been in my life and I stood alone. My mom even started to tell me again to get more tests done. I realize that people care but really they are starting to make me feel like a child. The thing is, I will never treat my children in such a condescending manner. To top it off, I physically feel like I am dying here. My head is pounding, I am dizzy, my left eyeball is so sore that I give myself stuns of pain when I look around. My eyes have difficulty converging on the same object at once, somewhat blurring. My lips and face are vibrating almost in constant tremor. Of course it would be difficult for anyone else to notice. My fingers are numb inside, so are my feet. I have no balance. My legs are extremely weak. I can't walk down stairs without both of my hands grasping the railing at the same time. Walking down, my legs just dangle in mid-air. Insomnia wakes me at 5am. My feet twitch and jar suddenly whenever they feel like it, especially when I lay in bed and I am pretty sure that I forgot something. Oh, yes, when I have a bath, like this morning, I leave a horizontal strip of greyish brown behind where I've been sitting. I have asked my husband's opinion too. I smell like sweet milk, like colostrum. In my book this is a common smell to those with chronic Mercury poisoning.

We get to the 'Chelation Centre' and a physician is there. He asks me how I am. I tell him that I am doing very poorly. I asked him if my urine test that Dr. Beattie sent away was in yet. He told me, "No." I was disappointed. I told him that I had a urine test done in Chatham for Mercury out of my own sheer ambition. I told him that I had the phone number and he told me he had a number himself. He got on the phone and told the man, he needed results as he had a very sick young nurse to take care of. The man told him, he didn't know how long the test would be pending. I was so down. Then the physician

118

brought me a tape to take home and listen to, to increase my knowledge of Mercury poisoning. I told him that I had already read much but that I would be happy to add to that knowledge. The whole time, I am thinking, "All I really want is some proof for these people so that they will give me the medication to get this garbage out of my brain." The physician came to see me later as I sat in my chair with intravenous E.D.T.A. going into my bloodstream. He told me that he was sorry. He told me to be patient and he touched my cheek and stroked it. I should not have listened to my friend Cindy. I should have gone with the feeling to go with that physician. Cindy thought he was weird. And so what if he looked different? This man has more compassion and time than Dr. Beattie. On my first day there, this man had passed me knowledge that Dr. Beattie probably wouldn't have been pleased he gave me. From the literature he gave me, I learned that the two oral chelating pills were the only way to capture the Mercury and get it out of one's system.

As I sat there, more knowledge was shared with me from two men who had severe angina. One man had his coronary artery 100% blocked and did not have angina anymore since he came every month for chelating. He had averted a coronary bypass operation. I asked Frank if his doctor sent him.

He laughed. He used to not be able to work but now he works ten-hour days again. His doctor refuses to acknowledge the success of chelating. He tells me that all provinces/states aren't like this. In Tennessee he believed that they made people have chelating before they would consider a bypass. I believe that Alberta has government coverage for chelating as well. These men see all this bypass and medication giving as moneymakers. They are chelating with the same medication as me but for different reasons. It pulls congested Calcium out of their arteries. Another woman, I performed Therapeutic Touch on. I had to offer T.T. to this lady. I could not ignore the direction I felt. Her left hand, where they tried to put her I.V. at as a first try, was swelling up with fluid. Since her chair was beside mine, after the nurse checked out her swelling and pushed on it to try to get it to deflate, I offered her Therapeutic Touch. She asked me questions and said she would mention it to her very sick niece who is in the hospital, I believe with Cystic Fibrosis, that some nurses in the hospital are trained to do it and Therapeutic Touch is endorsed by the College of Nurses; our governing body. I gave a little educational talk to her husband and another man too when they questioned me about it. Her husband asked me if I was qualified. "Yes, I am a Recognized Practitioner of Therapeutic Touch and have taken all the courses," I told him. I also shared a personal story about my husband's cramps and diarrhoea on last year's vacation, suddenly coming to an abrupt halt after I did T.T. on him, such that it surprised me. It surprised them too. I told them that T.T. decreases the frequency of pain medication, accelerates wound healing, accelerates bone growth in fractures and elicits a profound relaxation response. This of course is all while I feel very ill, but I am sitting, so it helps. Besides, being with these people cheers me up. When his wife asked me if T.T. was mind over matter, I told her, "No." I explained anyone could do it. It is about intention. And that it is non-denominational. It is based on working with universal energy. I told her that it fits with Einstein's theories. It is about all matter being made up of energy; some solid, some liquid and some gaseous states. I told her that the energy doesn't come from the practitioner, but through them. I told her I agreed with Rev. David Maginley, that it is God's gift to humanity, that we do this for each other. I am sure that there are fearful people who refuse to accept the power of human love. I personally would find this sad, if one would try to help their fellow human being and receive negativity. These people, I believe will not be the ones asking for T.T. They can mind their business because this is not the world; we live in. I am glad that the College of Nurses is on board, endorsing Therapeutic Touch. One of the nurses who taught me works at a Chatham hospital on patients receiving chemotherapy. I didn't intend to get into this, but back on my Mercury track. I managed to get to the bathroom with my I.V. and without falling over, but I still have my dad's cane so that helped. When I was getting it removed, since I was standing, I almost lost my balance and fell, but I didn't. I had requested to see Dr. Beattie. I had to talk to him about my need for oral chelators. In the morning in front of everyone I let him know how ill I was. I made sure he took me seriously. Now in the office, I talked to him and he said that he needed proof.

I persisted. I told him to watch my lips when I parted them to observe the tremor. He saw it and he saw it near my eye. He finally heard me and was going to call a London pharmacy as he had been out of stock of the meds he told me this last Monday. I thought to myself that he could have attained them by now if he tried sooner. Then I told him that I had the doctor's number for the M.D.S. laboratory in Chatham given to me by Paula. Paula had also given me the doctor's requisition number. He called. I watched and listened, figuring that the test would still be pending. Dr. Beattie hung up the phone and looked at me. He said no; the results were in. I was eager but a little afraid. He explained that a normal level of urine Mercury ranged from 0-5. Then he said, "Not that Mercury in one's urine is ever normal." Then he looked me in the eye and told me, "Yours was 18.5, very high!" I immediately started to tremble and cry; happy tears of course. What a release! This was the proof everyone else needed. God and I, we already knew I was poisoned. When Dr. Beattie proclaimed that this was the proof that I needed, I told him I already knew this down to the depths of my heart and my soul. Then he tried to tell me he thought so too. I could tell different, his faith wasn't in me; but at least now he would have been willing to give me the drug. I went to tell my mom. I held my arms out and told her that I needed a hug now. I couldn't get the drug in London, it was out of their stock, but I suggested Toronto since my mom reminded me that my dad was already there today. By talking with Dr. Beattie, I found out that there were only these two places that he had ever attained this drug; one pharmacy in London, the other in Toronto. I was still very ill, but I was happy. He asked me how I had gotten the urinalysis so promptly done. I told him that Monday before I went into the doctor's office, I said a prayer.

On the way home we listened to the tape lent to me by the physician. It even mentioned that in Germany, 85% of people with M.S. were cured after getting their amalgams out. The link I had pondered and concluded myself, but now my mom and I heard some proof. My mom apologized to me. I picked up my children at school. I immediately hugged them individually. I took them aside in the hallway and together thanked them for believing in me when absolutely no one else would. When my mom got me home, I checked the phone answering machine; my husband had left a message, so I called him back. I let him know with conviction and all the strength of my soul that the proof he needed, I had gotten. Then I told him that though I appreciated the thought of flowers, yesterday I had only needed his friendship and faith in me. I told him with how completely ill I was last night that the only flowers he would have needed to buy me would have been for my grave. I let out my pain with peace, confidence and strength. It felt good. I didn't mention the amount of times that I thanked God today, too many to count. I knew something was going to happen today. It was beyond my wildest dreams. I even called Wendy back as she finally returned my call. She left me a message when I was on vacation that she had had a dream about me. She told me today that she hadn't had a good night sleep since. I explained to her what had happened to me lately. Even though she confidently told me heavy metals weren't my problem and proclaimed it to my face several times, I never believed her. I listened to my inner self. I thanked her for what she did do for me. I told her there were no ill feelings, that was not who I was. She told me that I have to share and teach people, this I had a handle on too. My mom did not like that I spoke so long to Wendy because she wanted me to eat something more than I had today. Also, she thought I could have dropped dead in the intense heat of the sauna. But, as I told my mom, I was told when to get out, not by Wendy but by inner guidance. I do understand why my mom was worried. But all is forgiven. My trust may have to be earned by some; but faith in God, my children and my mom has never wavered. This proof for others; which I realize for some may never be enough, is the best birthday present that I could hope for. At least now I have human-acceptable proof when I say that I have chronic Mercury poisoning. Thank you God for being my sustenance! A world without true human support can be very tough.

It has been two weeks since I have written. Does that give any indication of how ill/poisoned I have been? If you know me and what has went on, it should. The last thing that I remember was telling Dr. Beattie how ill that I was and that I needed medication more than once per day. I told him this because I read it is more damaging to a person to not keep it constant in their blood stream. He agreed with my request. I had I.V. vitamin C at my request. My typing is not the best; the fingers are still numb inside but my feet, well. Two nights ago I was terrified out of my mind as the inside of my feet and legs were solidly numb, feet 100%. I guess that is the last time I am chelating and eat healthy meat spaghetti with garlic and take homeopathy for the first cold I had had in a year. Anyhow, I felt as close to depression as I'd ever felt. This is mostly because of the fact that people seem to make fun of me and/or do not care at all to see how I am. Doing Therapeutic Touch for a good half hour and reading spiritual literature, of course the best, being the Bible; where Jesus states, "Of course they hate you, they hated me. I am not of this world and neither are you." I understand the context of what I read and it comforted me. I also came across a Bible verse on the Internet, which talks about us being here to help one another. I only have to remember the written verse, I thought it was John but I can't find it.

To sum it up, I have gotten comfort from sleeping. I napped last Saturday. I have no idea how I made it to church that night as I spent the whole day in bed. But I had no feeling of implorement to cancel. I am so glad. I was well to sing and "On Eagle's Wings" yet! I got Dr. Beattie to order me D.M.P.S. instead. It took me a lot of work to get in touch with him and let him know my thoughts and what I was going through. He kept not calling me back. I am almost certainly his most ill patient. I kept at it and got him to order the medication from Toronto. I also got myself a dental appointment in Columbus, Ohio on April 8th and 9th with a reputable, famous dentist yet. He has a Cavitation ultrasound machine. The surgery to dispose of the toxic remains of my root canal on my jawbone will be on the 9th, if it shows as I think it should. In the meantime, I put D.M.S.A. on my grey gum. It turned pink in two days. My London dentist was surprised to see its betterment.

I told him that it didn't look this way two days ago. How can I sum up the most painful and difficult moment of my life? I could hardly walk at one point, after the meat, garlic and homeopathy. I know how I'll sum it up, going down stairs, preposterous. Two nights ago I fell, my knee just gave out. I didn't get hurt though. But to sum it up, there is certainly no shortage of suffering to offer UP. My mom sacrificed a lot for me out of her kindness and compassion. This was the only time that I have not been taking care of my children on a March break. The last two weeks have been a version of sheer and utter hell. But, as with pain, offering is the only decent purpose it has. So much happened, but at the moment it is lost. I can only share one moment, yesterday or the day before that I called out to God and told Him how incredibly much I love Him, I thanked Him for what He did for me on Oct. 15th, 2002 and my whole lifetime for that matter. I told God, "This time it's my turn to let you feel the depth of love I have for You." It made me cry.

CHAPTER 39

Help One Another

My right knee has given out several times since, making me fall, but yet I have never been hurt when I fell. Just today I realized that I still couldn't grasp how people cannot tell the pain and difficulty my body is giving me. Can't they tell my legs feel like heavy logs and that my feet are numb on their entire interior? As I said, "It gets worse if I have to eat out of my home, which is very rare." I basically have been driven around for two solid weeks. My right eye will start to go in a different vision field than my left and the dizziness and spinning will still show itself occasionally. I know when my face starts to tremble, it is time for the Alpha Lipoic Acid; it helps. To be honest I can't figure out how going down stairs is terrifying and so foreign. I can't even describe it! That is saying a lot. I saw the gynaecologist in London this week. He told me that my urine was very abundant in Mercury.

He asked me my symptoms. He believed. He offered me a neurologist; he wanted to make sure I got this metal out. I basically told him at this time, most doctors didn't know what to do with what I was experiencing and I showed him the drugs that I was taking. I asked him to have blood work done and he complied. I told him how he helped me by what he said to me last time and I thanked him for being who he was. I also got to tell him about my deductions. About why my iron was low in my blood work last month. It was close to 'anaemia.' I told him it had never been low in my life until the present and that I had figured this out by using my nursing manuals, realizing haemorrhage was not a reason and there were other sources; that Mercury would pull iron out of the blood. He agreed with me! I had a medical doctor backing me up. He point blank told me as he looked me in the eye that, "Yes indeed Mercury would pull iron out of the blood." I have another appointment with him. He wants to monitor me, even though he said it wasn't his specific field. I just love him. He was so supportive. He told me that I was doing a good job.

CHAPTER 40

A Supremely Gifted Dentist With An Incredible Heart

On the feast of St. Joseph, something amazing happened. I decided to call Dr. Estrabillo and check to see if I could get into see him sooner than the dentist in Ohio. I was inspired by how incredibly ill that I felt and how my life had ceased to exist for me. Also, I desperately wanted my root canal tooth out. I felt it a cause of toxin holding. I was amazed, well sort of; they had a cancellation the next day, sixteen hours later. I first said no; then got my husband's opinion if he could take me. Then my dad called to encourage me to do it. I knew this happened for a reason; I called to book it, not even knowing if surgery would be sooner with Dr. Estrabillo. I totally thought it impossible as he was booking into May. But I really wanted a 'Cavitat scan,' maybe a root canal tooth ripped out? Somehow, I was blessed. I even got my X-rays from the London dentist on the way to 'Ancaster' for 10am. I asked Scott what number of cavitations he thought that I had, out of four being the maximum possible. I told him that I hoped I wasn't right, but that I had four sights in mind.

As I talked with Dr. Estrabillo, he over time; began to see whom I was, how dedicated I was and how hard I had worked, for at least a year, to cleanse and figure out the problem. "You diagnosed yourself," he said. He was right; I did with God's help. During this time doctors such as Beattie heard me. Things seemed to happen. I want to do God's will. I want to help others. No one else need go through this garbage; be it the will of God. Dr. Roland Estrabillo was the first person that I had met in my life that credited his son for his learning and where he was at in his life. Someone who had this in common with me! And the Ohio doctor was his mentor and taught him. Then he told me, moments before my appointment that he cancelled a conference and could take me to do surgery on March 27th, 2002. That's next week! Yee Haw! You have no idea how happy you have made me, I thanked everyone and got to our vehicle and thanked God. I told my husband that God had His hand in today. The day clicked with ease and beauty. And believe me, I held onto nothing. At one point, I had given up that anything would happen with the 'Cavitat' or surgery with Dr. Estrabillo after I listened to him. But I figured that we had met for a reason, that there was a purpose, even if only that we share our stories with each other. Then he said he'd do the 'Cavitat.' It was not a picture of healthy jaws; there was only one almost completely decent area. And he talked to my husband about the support that I needed and the severity of my situation. God bless him! He's even a Eucharistic minister who has struggled with feeling alone. He's off the tribal path too like me. This is another confirmation from God that He is doing this.

CHAPTER 41

Understanding Heart Attacks

I finally got my 'anointing of the sick' by Father Joseph today. Boy, did I talk to him. I was laughing so loud and hard at one point; I know I freaked him out. But I am glad I can laugh, considering what I am going through. Mercury poisoning makes one dull, quiet, boring and unable to laugh. The oil he placed on my head smells and feels beautiful. And look at me, I am writing! Speaking of two years ago; I had a vitamin C-I.V. and the nurse stuck the I.V. needle in my artery, not my vein where it is supposed to be and let the fluid drip start. I asked her three times to pull it out because I felt horrible physically. My strength was gone completely; my chest hurt and my blood pressure was 58/13. She finally did pull the I.V. out. I physically felt like I was dying. Good thing my mom was sitting beside me. I kept living because I thought, "I can't die in front of my mother." I went to see Dr. Beattie immediately and while in his office, I saw a white light vision to my right side. He did an E.K.G. with no damage results. In my learned opinion, the E.K.G. was taken too soon after the incident. Though I left the office promptly, I had to make sure the nurse who did it to me was all right before I left. I cared about how she felt.

I went to 'Parks Blueberries' on the way home because I needed to get the babysitter a birthday present, as it was her birthday that day, even though I felt sick. I came up surprisingly behind the clerk as she was looking for something that I asked her for. "You just about gave me a heart attack," she said. This is confirmation.

I asked my M.D. for a blood test the next day. The blood test that I'd researched in my nursing manual on heart attacks that would show positive if a person had the test done the day after the heart attack. It's called 'Lactic Dehydrogenise.' My results came back a few days later and it showed that I did have a heart attack. I knew it. I drove to church the evening that I had the attack and asked for 'Last Rights' as I was feeling still very unwell and had pain around my heart. The priest told me at first that some people really do have heart attacks. I told him that I had but it was under different circumstances. He finally did give the sacrament to me and I am so grateful. I wrote a poem where the words just came to me late that evening, June 27, 2003. I was told to write what I received. It's copyrighted and it's entitled, "Love of God." "Love of God, deep within our heart and soul. Never doubt, never stray; know I'm with you every day. Love one another as I loved you. Truth of God is within you. The pain you suffer; the hurt, remorse; confide and offer, I'll chart your course. Your with-outs you know as sin. I come to tell you; **love** is with-in."

CHAPTER 42

Kind Aid and Knowledge

I'm continuing on health, but on different subjects. It is also unusual for me to supply gluten-free communion bread to my church by the 'Benedictine Sisters' in the U.S., but it's only 0.01% gluten. Their telephone number is (660)-944-2227. It just came out early in 2004 and is not supposed to touch regular communion bread, as this will make it contaminated. This communion bread is wheat based and is approved by Rome.

'Celiac Disease' often occurs (gluten intolerance) in Mercury poisoned individuals. You feel horrible; you quickly learn not to eat what makes you feel awful. 'Celiac Disease' only shows in about one-third of those who are blood tested for it; but they are still intolerant of sulphur foods/drinks and are ridden with 'Celiac Disease' even if their M.D. tells them they are not. Being Mercury poisoned; sulphur food makes me feel incredibly ill.

I also had medical tests: blood, stool and urine that went to 'Doctor's Data' in the U.S. The results went to Dr. D. Harper as he ordered them for me. I showed allergic to certain foods, the worst being eggs. This is common in Mercury poisoned people. I am also allergic to the common baker's yeast, brewer's yeast and tomatoes too. Also, in my results a systemic yeast infection showed when I had my blood taken by a woman registered to take blood. With my symptoms and research, I already knew I had this. Even my large intestine showed to have holes in it, what got through in my stool test showed the 'Leaky Gut.' Now I have proof but it's still not enough for my family. My dad even threatened Dr. Harper's job too.

Dr. Harper has been incredibly helpful. He knew I had parasites and had to work at disposing myself of them. He had unconventional laser treatment and since I've been to him; the severe, severe back pain is no more. I am so ecstatic in disposing of the pain. He is a chiropractor who does no bone cracking but insists on seeing x-rays that have been taken and previous chiropractic assessments.

CHAPTER 43

The Beginning of the Separation

Let me sum it up. On Aug. 20th, 2003 Scott called from work kindly and he closed with, "I want to have sex with you when I get home." I said, "I'm glad you find me good for something."

Scott said, "You're wrong, I find you good for nothing."

I was shocked and hurt. I told Daniel and Samantha in an appropriate way. I called my mom and said, "This is what he said, how are you going to stick up for him this time?"

As we were tucking the kids in at 7:30pm, I told him that I was hurt by what he had said. He denied ever having said it; he said that I was making it up. I was shocked once again. I was so hurt that the next morning, I had to go to mass at 8am.

Father Joseph's gospel reading was, "If you have trouble with someone, talk to them. If they don't listen, tell three people. If you still have trouble, tell the church." The reading resonated with me completely. I did the first two things. The gospel made me get through it. Thank you, God.

The week after Christmas 2003, Scott told me I'd have no money, he called at 10am. He said he and my dad would be coming to talk to me. They were upset that I had done alternative healing with 'Ayurvedic Doctors' and used the ion cleanse when there. This is when I knew that I needed to get out. A friend went with me to my current financer's office and nothing happened when I said that I needed money. My dad and husband had the same financer then. I went to C.I.B.C. and withdrew $200.00 X 3. My friend helped me figure this one out. I stayed at Wendy's house with her permission. On New Year's Day, 2004 I went to mass by myself. On Jan 9th, 2004 Scott came to Wendy's house. He came upstairs where I stayed and in front of her yelled, "You're dying! You're dying! Go to the hospital now with me, or I'm calling the cops." He did call the police. Wendy said that she'd go with me instead if I wished. He called the police off. Of course, I walked by myself. I held onto Wendy for the long distance walk, only for balance. My family members admitted me to the psychiatric ward with the M.D.'s help because I had an appointment with Bonnie Morey on Jan.10th, 2004 in Niagara-on-the-Lake. They didn't want me to go, so they locked me up with a M.D.'s help. I saw a psychiatrist because my dad and husband wanted to keep me captive and they talked my M.D. into it; the psychiatrist put me on 'schizophrenic' drugs, which would be fine if I had it. I got out after 10 days of hell, courtesy of my lawyer, Mr. Mitchell, attending the damaging family meeting. At the family meeting it was the case of competition between my dad and my husband. They both mocked my deep faith openly in front of the psychiatrist. They tried to make me crazy because of my deep faith. I wish that I had never shared my faith experiences with my husband or my mom. What a hurtful, emotionally damaging experience. They did this to me because they think that I'm bananas because I believe in something other than drugs, except my chelating drugs which they also think is crazy. All the medical proof of Mercury poisoning is futile. I have been told often that I know too much. Guess what, I also am invariably in tune with myself. I do things because I feel them, not think them. I just heard on T.V. this week that the drug "Zyprexa" causes diabetes. This is the drug that the psychiatrist put me on for no reason and he told me if I didn't take it by mouth, he'd inject me with it. Towards the end of hospital hell, I flushed pieces down the toilet because I felt too physically sick when I took it. I told a trusted nurse, working there, and she supported me doing this.

When I left the hospital to stay at my parents because I wouldn't go back to Scott, my dad told me to keep taking the drug. I answered, "No way; it makes me sick." When I arrived at the house with my mom, strong girl could not even make it up one stair. This was scary and the first time in my life that this ever happened.

Different people told me; I should sue my parents and my husband. What they did to me is not legal.

On the divorce paper handed to me by Scott's lawyer's representative on June 11th, 2004; it said that I was physically and MENTALLY unable to take care of myself. I despise this man for his evil lying. God sees it all. God help me from being judgemental. I know it angers you too, Lord.

CHAPTER 44

I Married Someone Like My Dad

On May 17th of 2005 my dad called in the evening and said, "You don't know what you are doing. You can't do anything right." He said that my head wasn't on straight because Scott and I agreed to sell the house. The "For-Sale" sign went up today because Scott and I agreed to sell the house. I got verbal assault from my dad. He said that I abandoned my family. Verbal abuse is not tolerable; neither is being a control-freak without a heart. I hung up on him twice. No one on earth deserves abuse.

My dad called and said that he was sorry for being so rough on me yesterday. Then once again, he told me that I abandoned my family and liked friends better. He offered me a ride to church Sunday. "No thanks," I said. It is emotionally damaging to be around him. My mom too seems to side with him, thinks my marriage should not end. Verbal abuse is O.K. with her too. My dad called the police on Larry Grineage with C.H.A.P.S., who drives for me. He is my friend and told me because he had to go to the police station. I had to answer the police too. My dad told Larry that I was incompetent. It's a good thing that Larry does not believe lies and truly is kind and helpful to me. I was assessed in Thamesville by Ike Lindenburger, S.W., M.Div. and he couldn't believe that this was done to me; me neither. My dad paid the woman, a nurse for the original assessment full of lies. I think that she thought me nuts because I was stupid enough to mention Mercury poisoning. She said that others dressed me, when they never did. The lies go on and on. She never even submitted her report to the guardianship board. This is a total lack of legality. She must have known that it was deceitful and was in it for the money. She said that I could get reassessed in six months, right at the start of her assessment. Not fun to be tormented and lied about. I paid Ike for the legal assessment. Ike told me how what the woman did lacked legality because it was devoid of proper submission.

He said that he's not afraid of my dad's threats, when I told him that I never gave his name as my dad has a reputation for threatening people. He told me to not be afraid. He said that he'd go to court for me. I still owe Ike $300.00; it's paid now. I dropped the power-of-attorneys before assessment as instructed. I went to my lawyer for this. I never used my power-of-attorneys for anything anyway. I always did my own stuff. I was just cut off from paying my lawyer, except for $1000.00. I still owe him $3000.00. I paid completely all owing funds this week, June 11/05. My mom refused to pay before. I asked her kindly four separate times when she asked me if I needed anything. My dad is still trying to control me. He even hated the power-of-attorneys that I chose. He sent them each very threatening letters. All he truly loves is money and control. He even told my mom once, "I love you but I don't respect you."

I left a message with my lawyer on May 18th that I want a restraining order done on my parents. They treat me like an infant that they want to control. No more! My dad does not treat me like a grown woman.

He's a control freak that says he loves me; I have never seen it. He loves money and control only.

I wrote my children's books on disc and typed them up; my dad over the phone said that I couldn't type. He is judgemental and thinks he knows it all and tells me what to do. I don't listen to ignorance. I know myself. He's trying to rule over me. Though I use a wheelchair, my dad is treating me like I'm a stupid child who is incapable of everything, even choosing my friends. The verbal abuse and trying to control me need to stop. It would make me happy to have a restraining order against my dad. He needs to leave me alone, so I can live my own life and not have people around me subjected to threats.

He thinks that I should not have a separation from my husband who works for him. You want to talk stupidity, I married a man who is verbally abusive like my dad, but at least he's easing up, my dad is the worst. When I could have used their compassion and kindness the most, it turned into "slam Pam."

My dad is verbally abusive to me. Just last week, Mary the real estate broker who runs 'Thamesville Manor' brought me to the tiny ranch house that I wanted to see on Victoria Ave. That night, my dad called at 7pm and said, "You saw a house on Victoria. I don't know what you're thinking. You can't do anything right."

I hung up on him twice. No one deserves the verbal abuse that he has given to me. I had to cry it out profusely, what he said to me. He has cut me up face to face a lot too. For a very long time, I don't want to be anywhere near him, even in the same vicinity. He treats me like I'm stupid and don't have a brain. I appreciate inheriting his intelligence and memory, but I would never abuse anyone like him.

No one would ever consider him anything but a wonderful, very smart businessman; but how he acts towards his daughter behind closed doors is abuse. The man has threatened my friends and even went to the police on a C.H.A.P.S. driver for no reason. I don't have my license and the man is seeking to take my transportation, which I am now paying for, away from me. He keeps telling me that friends mean more than family to me. Well, I would not choose friends that verbally abuse me. I had to have my competency reassessed; the woman who assessed me the first time told me that I could do this in six months. I legally paid for it and arranged for the assessment on my own. I was eager to tell my parents the results, after the torture that I unnecessarily went through, the first thing out of my dad's mouth was, "Who did it?" Even after I told him before that it was legally done.

In the fall of 2003 Scott told me that his mother and brother were so much more religious than me.

He said months later in the spring, "What, do you think you're God?"

Verbal abuse was not rare, it happened at least every week. My husband would not let me see the kids without supervision. He told me that it was, 'Children's Aid' doing this to me. I never should have mentioned at the 'Woman's Shelter' that my husband once hit Daniel with a belt. I told her that this was once. He did it no more.

But he turned his anger toward me and played phoney with 'Children's Aid.' Even my physician said it sounded like malarkey. It is resounded finally.

"No more," Scott finally said on June 13th, 2005.

The time is up. I endured tremendous suffering. Angelic seeming to others Scott, had tried to prevail. I don't want to be anywhere near to my dad, even in the same vicinity. He treats me like I'm stupid and don't have a brain. I appreciate inheriting his intelligence and memory, but I would never abuse anyone like he does.

CHAPTER 45

Yeast (A Parasite) and Mercury Go Together

Parasites show as tiny white eggs in my urine. In my colon cleanse a massive amount showed in my stool after the colon cleanse last Wed., Oct 5th, 2005. The nurse-cleanser said one month ago that it was the first time that she did not see little white things in my stool. I guess that 33 day fast on just liquids worked. I did it to give my intestines a break so that they'd heal easier and I did not take vitamins so that I wouldn't feed those obvious parasites. The colon cleanse having the results it did made me happy. Last year when I had colon cleanses, she saw shiny metal pieces coming out in my stool.

Mercury is the world's second worst poison and yet they put it in people's teeth. Even the 'World Health Organization' says that 87% of Mercury poisoning in people comes from their teeth.

I've learned from Dr. Cutler that autoimmune disease; physicians like to think people are stuck with forever, but Mercury poisoning mimics this and it's curable. Do physicians know what yeast and parasites appear like in people's brains? I don't think that they learn this in medical school. It would be good if they learnt more about nutrition too. Food can be damaging if it is deficient in nutrients and subjected to herbicides and pesticides. I am so grateful that M.D.'s prescribe D.M.P.S. and D.M.S.A. But I do have access to the D.M.S.A. in a U.S. company now. Myself, I prefer how I feel taking the D.M.P.S. I did chelating on the children, as I did not want them to go through in any way what their mommy is going through. Mercury crosses the placenta; this is how it gets into the children of a poisoned mother. I did chelating with D.M.S.A., as it is the only one specific and approved in the U.S. for children. The physician prescribed it for me and prescribed A.L.A. pertaining to their body weight also. I gave them Alpha Lipoic Acid (A.L.A.) every four hours, three days per week for seven weeks. I made sure that they ate no sulphur for the three days chelating because sulphur slows chelating down and I awoke them at night on schedule to keep it in their bloodstream. I monitored them closely and asked them how they felt because I am their mother who adores them and a registered nurse. They felt great and the results of chelating showed in their urine test that I got and sent away to the U.S. laboratory when the family M.D. kindly prescribed the urinalysis for heavy metals for my children. My daughter's urine, I took after the first chelating session with D.M.S.A. and Alpha Lipoic acid. The result showed Mercury and a high Arsenic level. Dr. Beattie was shocked at how high the Arsenic was for a five-year-old child. I have since had to find a new M.D. as my now ex threatened Dr. Beattie's medical license because he prescribed for the kids; Dr. Beattie wants nothing more to do with me because of this. I can get D.M.S.A. myself now in the U.S., so I wish I could do it all over again and not have to involve a M.D. in the situation. It has been rough but I get through the brutality because I know that God sees it all.

LET'S WORK TOGETHER AND HELP ONE ANOTHER; THE UNNECESSARY, UNSEEN SUFFERING NEEDS TO STOP!

In May of 2005, a physician looked in my ears with an otoscope because I asked him and he said, "Your ears are full of yeast."

On June 9th of 2005 I saw E. Mac Rae, M.D., an otorhinolaryngologist (ear, nose, throat specialist), who examined my right ear and suctioned it. I knew what it was and never mentioned it, but I asked him what he thought? He said, "Undoubtedly, it is a fungal infection and you're taking the right stuff." I am so glad that I researched and asked a M.D. for the 'Terbinafine' a.k.a 'Lamisil.' I am glad that God guides me to know so much. I want to help others. I have been blessed. Dr. MacRae wants to see me again at Newbury Hospital on June 28th/05 to vacuum my right ear again. He comes from London, ON. I have been so blessed as to meet two doctors with hearts, listening ears and intelligence. I am glad that they help the woman that is so outside of the box.

On June 10th of 2005 I saw Dr. Bell the naturopath and he said that my ear is still angry. He said that a severe fungal infection, as I have, is not common. My immune system is damaged. I knew this. He agreed with me and said it was no irony that the infected side is the same side that the Mercury draining root canal was on.

On Oct. 5th, 2005 I got my ears suctioned and examined by Dr. MacRae again. God bless him. He said that the fungus was showing no more, the only thing coming out of my ear was wax. He made me laugh and that continues because of what he said. When the nurse asked if I was allergic to anything, he said in a couple of minutes, "Yes, she's allergic to sexy men."

I've learned by Andy's education on "Amalgam Illness" that you'll get rid of the yeast when you get rid of the Mercury. I've learned that Mercury damages all the cells in one's body and it is thus, very damaging to the immune system.

CHAPTER 46

Effects On The Children

The kids treated me like I was garbage today. I forgive them. I know who is teaching them. Daniel gave me condemnation for having vitamins and told me that they threw them all in the garbage at the border after they had to wait a long time. I, thus, asked Scott who was teaching the kids this? Only today Scott told me that Daniel was there on a weekday when I was getting treatment for toxic shock. I was getting 'Septicaemia' treatment on Mar. 1st, 2004. Septicaemia (blood poisoning) had hit me on Feb. 29th, 2004. He denied it once, I called him on it again when he was in my bedroom, I told him that it was just Scott and my parents who were there when they crossed the border and my D.M.P.S. which is worth over $1000.00 and my vitamins got thrown in the garbage. Scott then said, "I think Daniel was there." He now is not speaking the same way.

On November 17th, 2005 I asked my daughter how she felt about what mom and dad are going through i.e. the separation and divorce. She said, "Bad" when I asked her how she felt, "Good or bad?" She didn't want to speak to me about it on her own.

Daniel has cooked on the stove when he is home alone after school. He hits his sister also. This scares me that a ten year old does this. It is dangerous and not legal and bothers their mother. I offered to Scott yesterday, Jan. 15th, 2004, that I would watch them after school. I am with Samantha on Tuesday only for her violin lessons, which I pay Chantelle for teaching. This is with Samantha's desire to continue learning when I asked her. In my opinion this is not enough supervision for children.

CHAPTER 47

Deep Faith Wins Over Poisoning

I watched "Touched by an Angel," today and I heard this song; I'm still singing it. It resonated with me, it happened to me and I'm comforted by the truth of the song. I gave Him my life and I only wish to do His will. No wonder that I love to sing it.

"FOR SUCH A TIME IS THIS, I WAS PLACED UPON THIS EARTH, TO HEAR THE VOICE OF GOD AND DO HIS WILL."

God spoke to me with clairaudience again on August 3rd, 2005 at 2:20pm. I was told to document what I heard and I was surprised to get the information. He said to me, "The best is in all of you. Follow Me!"

On August 24th, 2005 I spoke to Angie, she did ancient Egyptian work on me previously and said she didn't know what was doing it but the damage in my body was in my thyroid, pituitary gland and my large intestine. I knew it; Mercury has these physiological effects on the human body. She got her own idea and checked me for M.S. three times over. She said it kept coming up that I didn't have it; not even a hint or a minuscule amount. I said that I already knew this, but it was nice to have confirmation. This is another agreement. Dr. Um felt the same way, that it was poisoning doing this to me, so does Dr. Bell. "Oh, I have glorious naturopaths. I am so blessed to have others believe in my true self." God spoke with clairaudience to me this Monday morning, August 29th, 2005 and said, "Keep doing what you're doing. You were severely Mercury poisoned, your parents will get what they deserve from Me for what they've done to you."

Today is September 11th, 2005. Reverend Peter A. Black baptized me today. Peter is an incredible man with beautiful kindness. He shares God's love, as man should. It's a dream come true! I have been wishing to have baptism for over a year, not christened like I was traditionally baptized as an infant. I did ask the Catholic Church if they would baptize me again. The answer I received was, "No, you said you were baptized as an infant. That's it." The baptism that I received today was as Jesus taught; full immersion that causes purification. The Holy Spirit spoke to me through clairaudience on the way home in the van with Sadie and Mike. They have blessed me, are my spiritual sister and brother and drove me to 'Watford' for baptism in Scott's indoor pool.

The Holy Spirit said to me with clairaudience after just leaving the city of Watford, "You did the right thing. It allows Me to get closer to you and create a true unity of the Trinity within you."

Today is Oct. 10th, 2005 Sadie and Mike came for a visit. At the end of their visit, I asked if they'd mind looking at my eyes and tell me if they saw a difference. They were amazed; they said that the specks they remembered were gone. I asked them the color and they said the outside was blue. I was born with blue eyes. They changed to green in Grade 3 after I had a tantamount of amalgam fillings placed in my mouth. I'm detoxifying what doesn't belong and my natural color is coming back.

Today is Oct.11th, 2005. When getting ear candling done yesterday as I requested it because I said that I had a lot of pain in the right ear; I had a tremendous amount of wax come out of that ear, just like two days before.

It's November of 2005. I spoke to Mary the 'Vibrational Consultant.' She said, "Don't take 'homeopathy' when you're on 'Choming essences.' It's too much for the body to take."

I am getting rid of the parasites. The little white eggs aren't as proficient in my urine and after I defecate. After my colon cleanse, Carolyn said that the tiny white things are only visible when my 'Cecum' empties. This is a healing change for the better. I am taking garlic capsules now to keep yeast at bay and to get rid of parasites. I am also taking silver water and Oregon extract as a natural antibiotic too along with garlic. I have stopped the garlic now. I feel very ill on it. Such it is with Mercury poisoning, you can't tolerate sulphur foods.

After having Toxic Shock Syndrome begin last year on Feb. 29th, 2004 and it almost killed me, I must make sure that the gram-negative 'Staphylococcus Aureus' is dead. Having I.V. 'Plasmaphoresis' at Harper Hospital in Detroit three times, I found helped me. I had the appointment booked for 'Plasmaphoresis' on Mar. 2nd, 2004; where they said how sick I looked, took my vitals and did blood work immediately getting the results quickly of my incredibly high white blood cell count. If not for their caring and knowledge, I may not be here. The M.D. in emergency told me when I told him that I told my mom that I felt like I was dying, he said, "Good thing you got here when you did, you probably would have." I had a high fever, a very rapid pulse, high blood pressure and a speedy respiratory rate. I told my mom about feeling like I was dying at 1pm on Feb. 29th, 2004 and she didn't believe me, even though all I did was sleep and couldn't walk to the toilet and my bowels were just going unexpectedly for the first time in my life. My mom said, "It's just M.S." Just like my husband said to the staff at the Chatham hospital. They believed him, it did not seem to matter what the patient said or felt. Even the border guard in Detroit asked me if I needed an ambulance, as I looked so sick to her. I said that I just needed my husband to drive me to the hospital right away. Now my mom is blaming 'Plasmaphoresis.' I told her that I never stayed in the hospital for it, so I could not see one getting 'Staphylococcus Aureus,' the unclean hand illness from that, but when they stuck me on the Psychiatric Ward, I had to stay locked up in hospital for ten days of unnecessary treatment that started on Jan. 9th, 2004 before I got my lawyer in. This was damaging to my immune system. I didn't need this as Mercury weakens the body and thereby, the immune system. I'm positive that the poison is losing.

On Oct. 14th, 2005 my dad said that he would pay for the van that I had already bought. It has an automatic wheel-chair lift. They were asking $15,000.00 for this mint condition, 1994 Dodge Caravan with only 56,000 km on it. I offered $10,000 for it, but we agreed on the price of $11,000.00 plus applicable taxes. I got it in London, thanks to Larry's knowledge, research, advice and friendship.

There is healing from Mercury poisoning. It has been an incredible journey of faith and trust in God. The van payment, I am extremely grateful for. This was the evening. The morning of this day, I was not so impressed. Dr. Strobelle said that he talked to Dr. Beattie and they both think that I am in denial. It does not seem to matter how severely poisoned a human is, even if they urinated Mercury. The doctor does not agree with my knowledge and opinion; that it's very dangerous chelating someone while they still have Mercury amalgams in. I've learned otherwise from Andrew Cutler, PhD. He knows because he has been through it. He says that it does not show necessarily high levels of Mercury in a severely, chronically poisoned person. M.D.'s don't learn this in school; they won't know that things exist beyond the drug happy world unless they live it. Stop the labelling. The only thing believed is M.S. in a faulty M.R.I. Do M.D.'s know what yeast, parasites or Sims Virus 40 look like in the head or bloodstream? What about blood flukes? My 'Vibrational Consultant' diagnosed me with this. What about tapeworms? I had several alternative healing practitioners actually diagnose that I had one. But now after a 33 day fast with no vitamins, it's gone. I saw the mother tapeworm's head come out in my stool and with the 'Vibrational Consultant's Assessment' what was a 9 (10 being the highest level) came down to a 4 and now it is gloriously at 0 (meaning non-existent.) This is coming from me, a woman who feels a lot better taking D.M.P.S. appropriately with Lipoic Acid in order to keep it in her bloodstream.

December 16th, 2005; I am so incredibly happy today. Daniel said that he'd play "Panis Angelicus" on piano for my web site if I pay him. He has learned about life being only about how much money you have, so I understand the example. I am just ecstatic because my gifted boy said that he would play the piano, which he always loved, and this made him happy until my family and ex forced him, then he quit. I am thankful, God is watching over us. Samantha said that she would accompany him on violin if allowed practice time. This young, young girl was gifted for violin and loved it. My ex forced her to stop.

On November 26th, 2005 severe pain began on the right side of my neck. I couldn't even turn my head slightly to the right side and not experience severe, severe pain. So, I did not move my neck even slightly. On November 28th, 2005 I told Dr. Strobele that the pain was very severe until I began chelating with Lipoic Acid and D.M.P.S. that Monday morning. He said that people with arthritis are immediately pain-free chelating. He said that the relief that I felt was not atypical with chelating.

On December 4th, 2005, I watched my D.V.D. of, "What The Bleep Do We Know?" with Sadie and Mike. The point of the movie that crossed my mind now is in Quantum Physics too, people create how they are physically by what they think in their brain. Also, other peoples' thoughts about them physically create the outcome. This was hitting the nail on the head. When getting a M.R.I. test, my parents thought it, the hospital staff; I'm sure thought M.S. too. It does not seem to matter what the individual thinks or feels. Even with the 'Bio signature' test that says there is not even a hint of Multiple Sclerosis in me, judgemental people don't believe this ancient test.

December 12th, 2005; I paid in full for Sadie to get her amalgam with Mercury crown out too. She was for the dentistry with Dr. Estrabillo and was shocked at how horrible her teeth looked. She had five amalgam fillings, not three as she thought she had. She insisted on seeing me before the dental work, though I said that I'd pay for it weeks before. She did say that she'd pay me back. She needed to have me say it to her face again that I'd pay for the work to be done. As Jesus said, "Love one another as I have loved you." I asked Sadie and Mike if they'd buy a big jug, they could fill it from my water system and drink the purest water to help both of them health wise. I am so happy that they brought me to Cheryl's and they bought organic eggs, which I recommended for Sadie to eat since with four amalgams left, she can't use the chelating drugs yet. They bought organic lamb too.

December 16th, 2005—I let my dad into my house with my children as my parents bought me a 'Full Spectrum' light, which I had wished for. It mimics natural sunlight. This is the only light that does this. It's an early Christmas present and my dad placed it in my bedroom as I asked for it to be there. This is a nice change. My children tell me that my eyes are blue when I ask them the color they see. I am detoxifying and the color that I was born with is thus, returning. Yesterday afternoon, Judy and Carol visited me. We prayed for Ellen's son Brian and I led the prayers. We also prayed for Rick, that he would be guided and brave enough to get assessed by Dr. Estrabillo and get the Mercury amalgams and root canals out of him. Judy and Carol are blessed sweethearts and faith filled friends.

Carol even bought two of my angel books. She was inspired to give one to a woman that came to her mind and heart. My Webmaster, the kind and knowledgeable computer expert, came by yesterday and will return today. He is setting up my website. I already had Lori from Florida request to see my website, when running. She would like to see my books that she may purchase, if she likes them. Today, January 6th, 2006 my mom came by kindly with rice milk but told me that eating bananas would be good for me and all the nutrition that I need is in food. She also blames me for living in the past and does not see why I choose to divorce a verbal abuser, even though he handed me the divorce papers first. She blames lawyers. She thinks that his lawyer makes him do things. The client does only what he/she wishes is my understanding. But, I'm easy to blame. Marie says that divorce turns God off.

I told her that the annulment was going through and that verbal abuse does not please our Lord and Savior. He knows that humans are to truly love and support one another. Let's do His will.

I am taking Basil, Kelp, 'Three-Lac' with Milk Sugar and some 'Stevia' for taste in the most purified and oxygenated water to combat Simian Virus 40. This virus came in the Polio vaccine. It supposedly stopped in 1963 but considering my symptoms and the fact that the pure air cleaner turned up on its own, the moment that I sat beside it in my wheelchair, made me wonder. This was the moment that I took my second time drink of kelp, basil and 'Three-Lac' in the best water. This was telling me that my body needed cleaning. I had unexplained, profuse diarrhoea today, January 19th, 2006. My body is cleansing. Simian Virus 40, I've researched and learned can be absorbed by the fetus or during childhood from a parent. I am sensitive and weak due to Mercury poisoning. I have a vacation booked to 'Our Lady of Lourdes' in France on May 9th, 2006. As of yesterday, Jan. 19th, Ellen says she'll go with me. My mom said that she'd pay for both of us. What an incredible blessing and change. I had planned to go by myself as I could afford it. I mailed Ellen's deposit today and talked to Norman who is the head of the 'Lourde's Center' in Boston, Massachusetts, U.S.A.

I talked to my mom on January 19, 2006 and told her that when watching 'Salt and Light' on satellite that it was stated that Jesus chose the ordinary, average man to be his apostle and continue His work. This should help her to understand the importance in herself, as she so often says that she's good at nothing and has no talents. Dealing with this Simian Virus 40 causes there to be tiny white floaters in my urine after I cleanse when I use my 'Pure Charge' machine in my bath water. I immerse my whole body including my head under water with earplugs in. I stay in for half an hour as instructed. I am orally chelating with D.M.P.S. and Alpha Lipoic Acid. I am chelating every other week to dispose of Mercury and Arsenic right now.

Dr. Bell worked on me intravenously Tuesday, February 14th, 2006. He gave me glutathione separately, Vitamin C and Vitamin B-12. Usually my left venous side is the best, but he discovered that it is overworked and needs cleaning. My Valentine's gift was that the I.V. went in my left arm and it worked, this was miraculous. I told Dr. Bell that when I had a bath with magnesium 'Epsom salts' the night before and a bath with the 'Pure Charge' the night before that; that there was a blackish, brownish ring around my head area only. I was fully submerged with earplugs on. He said that it sounds like metal coming out of me. I agree, I thought the same thing when I saw it.

Today, February 18th, 2005, my surrounding bathing area was clean with the 'Pure Charge.' My dad came over and said he'd bring a T.V. from the house and a DVD as I requested. My mom on the phone did not impress me as she thinks my daughter should be in English, not French Immersion. I knew this before but she is showing her true colors.

My parents are surprisingly being kinder than ever. I can still hear that they don't know me or believe in me. My mom heard me on my disc singing "Panis Angelicus" while Marilyn played the organ. She remarked that I always sang that song. I told her that I know the meaning of the Latin words and that's why it means so much to me. They also don't believe that their daughter is fighting severe, chronic Mercury poisoning. I had tonnes of medical proof, but it's not enough proof for some people. I love them for who they are; it's their learning journey.

Today is March 16th, 2006. What an incredible, blessed day. Beth came to teach my good friends from St. Ursula's choir about the natural benefits of the strongest magnets and the highest quality of water. Jim, Sheila and Agnes care about helping themselves and others without drugs. Beth gave them magnetic insoles, 'Jade Greenzymes' and a water unit to bring home and try. If they find the benefits in themselves, it sounds as if they will join the company to receive wholesale prices and be the first people under me. This would be wonderful. My true desire to help others is coming true.

I am taking 'Diabetaguard,' twice daily. I ordered and received it yesterday. It comes from the U.S. It is a natural supplement to get the body to make its own 'insulin.' Diabetes runs in my family, my dad's mom had it in her early forties, had gangrene and died shortly after. With each of my dad's brothers having it, I did not need to be on a psychiatric ward unnecessarily and forced to take "Zyprexa," a medication that has been researched and found to cause diabetes. I know how I feel, I understand and I am learning more than I ever intended by living it. God is guiding me and I am thankful.

I have researched and learned that I am 'Hypoadrenal,' also. That's why my blood pressure is so very low. Low cholesterol causes this. This happens in Mercury poisoning. First the cholesterol is very high for no reason, then for no reason it is now extremely low. This causes the thyroid to not function, as it should also. I am healing this naturally too. Glory, glory, halleluiah!

I had my stool sample with the giant white piece sticking out of it with the help of the order by Dr. Bell, my naturopath. The result showed nothing, but as Dr. Bell says, yeast, which we know I have, is not tested for. On May 26th, 2006 I told Dr. Bell that when I had a colon cleanse this week that Carolyn said yeast was coming out. She said my symptoms of very itchy eye; nose, head and body were typical with yeast infection. Dr. Bell felt the same. I wasn't surprised as I am taking a yeast killing formula from the U.S., which contains coconut oil called 'Monolaurin.' Dr. Glen Bell is a blessing and I let him know this. I am grateful my mom paid for my visit to him and thus what I purchased under his advice.

May 20th, 2006; I am once again not impressed by my mom. She said M.S. which one man was diagnosed with they cured at 'Lourdes.' I was so blessed to go to this place in France. What a wonderful, faith filled journey with others who have deep faith. I am so lucky that I was able to solo at mass time and again with Norman's and Fr. Normand's help.

I am outside of the box and people like labels. They won't look beyond. Mercury poisoning is not believed even if one has proof. This battle is akin to climbing a mountain, not a hill, as I have learned. I am incredibly grateful for the kind, rare understanding of one other person. I am going to redo my singing of "Panis Angelicus" with Christine Wilcosz-Thompson, this music is on my web site too. I asked because I believe it to sound better if I had a chance to practice it with her before the recording. I have an appointment booked on Friday, June 2nd, 2006 for a Full Body Digital Iriscope. I booked this now because my eyes are showing the change to the blue eye color I was born with. Yeast is horrible. My right ear is severely painful; God's love gets me through it all.

Let's get together and help one another. The unnecessary, unseen suffering needs to stop. My life has been one of suffering, healing, learning, faith and a desire to help others.

IRLEN SYNDROME—
READING
IS NOT EASY FOR
EVERYONE

Irlen Syndrome is a hidden mask worn by many children and adults alike. Reading has never been easy for them. But the person with Irlen Syndrome, approximately 10-15% of the population, does not realize that the rest of the world sees the page differently. The brain does not accurately perceive the printed word on the page. The words are distorted.

White paper is the main culprit. Fluorescent lighting is troublesome too. Often, the first minutes reading are manageable; then distortion and fatigue set in. Comprehension may be affected. Spelling can be difficult; b's and d's may be confused, portions of letters are sometimes not seen. Or, as in my son's case, the space between words may not be seen. It is rare that people have identical Irlen Syndrome symptoms. One commonality is that they don't enjoy reading.

Irlen Syndrome was discovered only in the 1980's. Testing for Irlen Syndrome is not part of school or medical testing. Though its discovery is recent, the T. V. show 60 Minutes provided information about it in 1988.

A trained professional easily solves the problems created by Irlen Syndrome. They follow a full testing protocol in order to find the best combination of colored overlays (transparent colored sheets that sit atop of white paper) for the individual. This is the first step. Lenses can be the last step. These additions change the person's reading ability. Therefore, schoolwork can be easy. Thus, comfort comes. Behavior is modified as well.

My son Daniel inspired me, to use color behind the printed word of my children's books so that many may find their reading easier. My son has Irlen Syndrome.

I was led to this in January of 2003 when my very gifted boy criticized himself by saying how stupid he was. He cut himself up brutally. I never could figure out why such a smart child had great trouble reading and hated learning to read. I believe that everything in life happens for a reason. When a Certified Irlen Syndrome Screener found the best color for him to use, my son quit fidgeting profusely while he was reading. He calmed down instantly and the space between words he saw again. If I hadn't taken him to get tested by a trained Irlen Syndrome professional, I never would have known that words ran all together for him.

Now my son has cool, blue-grey colored glasses to wear to school. They look like sunglasses. Believe it or not, my son has a mild form of the syndrome. Fortunately, I discovered this when he was young. Therefore, he will not find paperwork difficult when he matures. A key element is that he needs his family and teachers working together to support him and each other. Let's work together and help one another. The unnecessary, unseen suffering needs to stop.

Book by Helen Irlen is "Reading By The Colors—Overcoming dyslexia and other reading disabilities through the Irlen Method." ISBN 0-89529-9826 If your child is falling behind in reading and schoolwork, even math and music notes can be distorted; please call a Certified Irlen Syndrome Screener or a clinic. You'll be changing your child's future and helping the ones to come. This syndrome is genetic and runs in families.

Written and researched by: Pamela Elizabeth Lacek, R.N.

For more information, talk to:
Adele Francis-Director of Irlen Service Canada 1-800-934-7536
irlen@cyberus.com

AUTOBIOGRAPHY

I received the top of my class female award in grade eight. I was a painfully shy girl, as is common with Mercury poisoning. This did an about face when my amalgams were removed. I had a job at McDonald's beginning at age fifteen and lasting for almost three years. I was employee of the month once during this time.

I am a registered nurse who graduated at the very top of my class of about eighty people. The Victorian Order of Nurses hired me just after my graduation in 1994. I took a leave when pregnant as I had severe morning sickness with my son, which didn't stop after three months. He was born in September of 1995. I quit my nursing job, as I desired to be a full time, stay-at-home mother. I became pregnant again and had my daughter in 1997, one week and two years after my son. I raised them virtually by myself.

I was at a Woman's Shelter in 2003 due to verbal abuse and I took the kids with me.

I wrote a children's book in 1996 and 1998. They were published in Canada in 2006. One is on hand washing for kids because I am a nurse and wish to make simple illness prevention fun and easy for children, it is for ages five to twelve. The second book is about guardian angels and is for grades seven, eight and high school age. I illustrated it by water-color myself. My first children's story was published in the U.S. in the year 2000 in Guide magazine. It is entitled, "Locked Up Alone." It is non-fiction and my dad's childhood story when he was thought to have tuberculosis but this proved otherwise; he had swallowed a Dutch dime.

My children's books are called, "Germs Under Arrest" and "An Angel In My Room." My adult autobiographical book is called, "Mercury Poisoning and Deep Faith." I published this book because my deepest desire is to help others; they need not go through what I went through.

My life has become; live and learn. I am a vocalist. Christine Wilcosz-Thompson played, "Panis Angelicus," as I requested and I sang it for this website *www.rnhealingarts.com*. I have started a company called "RN Healing Arts." I am a book writer and illustrator. My two books have M.D.'s, a nurse beside myself, different denomination of religions and teacher quotations on the back covers. I have become a nutrition expert as I have lived with food allergies, which are common in Mercury poisoning. I have medical testing to prove all of this and a company in the U.S. to recommend. I have become a well-learned chelating expert. I can provide D.M.S.A. (which chelates Lead and Mercury) to others for chelating and I recommend a great book too by a P.H.D. who's lived it also.

CONTACTS

Dental Amalgam Mercury Syndrome International (DAMS)
Contact websites; *www.dams.cc* OR *www.noamalgams.org*
Telephone number: 1-800-311-6265

Andrew Hall-Cutler, PE, PhD
Telephone number: (425)-557-8299
Website: *www.noamalgams.com* Email: AndyCutler@aol.com

For incredible health naturally, contact *www.achew.com*
I bought my 'Pure Charge' machine from him.

Angie Spizzirri—health consultant, works using the most helpful ancient Egyptian dowsing also. She lives in Toronto, Ontario and can work long distance. Her telephone number is (416) 464-7463; Cell (416) 509-2148. She is incredible and I highly recommend her.

'Metagenics' products I sell to the clients of my business. I have become a partner to the 'Metagenics' business because I am a registered nurse who has a deep desire to help others. They produce the best natural vitamins, minerals, amino acids, essential fatty acids and high cholesterol healing natural medicine. Website: *www.metagenics.com*

I am a member of the 'Nikken' corporation and sell their products or help to make others a part of the business so that they get their products wholesale. They have the best in magnetic products, even mattresses. Their magnets are the highest quality. Magnets in a drug store or other stores don't get near the quality. Magnets heal the body from pain and are part of the earth's core; we need to bring them closer for benefits. Their website is: *www.nikken.com*

I also am a member of 'Mannatech,' you can be too. Their 'Ambrotose' is patented and is revolutionary in helping people. It is food also.
Website: *www.mannatech.com*

Cell Phone E.M.F. Harmonizer by 'BioPro. It lasts for the life of your cell phone. It has been medically proven to prevent brain tumors. Website: *www.bioprotechnology.ca*